HEALING HERBS
From
Your Kitchen

Mama Prepper

CONTENTS

1	Aloe Vera	4
2	Anise	8
3	Basil	12
4	Bay Leaves	17
5	Beans	20
6	Broccoli	23
7	Caraway Seeds	28
8	Carrots	31
9	Cayenne	34
10	Chives	43
11	Cinnamon	47
12	Cinnamon and Honey	50
13	Cloves	53
14	Coffee	56
15	Cilantro	61
16	Dill	61
17	Fennel	65
18	Garlic	72
19	Ginger	75
20	Green Tea	78

21	Marjoram	81
22	Onion	86
23	Oregano	90
24	Parsley	96
25	Radish	101
26	Rosemary	105
27	Sage	110
28	Summer Savory	114
29	Tarragon	119
30	Thyme	123
31	Tomato	128
32	Turmeric	135

1

Aloe Vera

Aloe Vera is one of the most versatile and useful skin remedies available. Here is a list of what Aloe Vera can be used to treat: acne, allergic reactions, athlete's foot, blisters, burns, eczema, fungicide, hemorrhoids, herpes sores, insect bites & stings, itching skin, poison ivy, psoriasis, rashes, rosacea, scalds, scars, shingles, sores, sty, sunburn, hives, vaginal infections, warts, wounds, wrinkles.

Anytime damage is done to the skin, Aloe Vera can begin the healing process.

Grow your plant in a pot on the porch, where it can get a lot of sun. If you live in a cold climate, bring your plant inside during the winter, but place it in a sunny window. Because it only needs to be watered once every week or two, it is very easy to care for.

The way to use Aloe Vera is easy too. Just cut the leaf off at its base, slit it lengthwise across the width of the leaf to harvest the gel.

Aloe Vera has been used for:

- Facials
- Hair Conditioner
- Skin irritations, burns, skin conditioning

- Analgesic
- Fungicide
- Gastrointestinal Issues

Facial Cleanser

For a soothing facial, use two parts Aloe Vera gel to one part honey, apply to face, let dry for 20 minutes, then wash off with clear water. It gives the skin a nice toned feeling.

It is gentle enough you can even remove your eye makeup with it.

Because Aloe Vera also has anti-bacterial properties, it works great applied on acne. Just smooth the gel all over the face, then rinse with clear water. The anti-bacterial effects in the gel fight the germs that continue your acne problem.

Hair Conditioner

Aloe Vera can be used as a hair conditioner, a scalp conditioner, and to help defeat dandruff. For dandruff and other scalp conditions, just massage the gel right into the scalp and let it sit for a couple of minutes before rinsing. You can replace your hair conditioner with the gel. Rub some of the gel onto your wet hands and smooth it over your wet hair, especially on the ends. Let it sit for a couple of minutes before rinsing it out.

Skin Irritations

Aloe Vera's anti-bacterial action also makes it work well for burns, cuts and sores. It also helps prevent scarring.
Do you have a rash of any kind? If you have ever endured a case of hives, be in misery no longer. Apply Aloe Vera to the affected skin. This also includes eczema, psoriasis, rosacea, allergic reactions and herpes outbreaks.

A Note on Eczema

Eczema is a balance issue. If you have this condition, your body is out of balance, and you need good nutrition to put it right again. So please understand that while Aloe Vera will ease your condition, it will not cure it.

Pregnant? Apply Aloe Vera to your stretching belly skin daily. It helps prevent stretch marks.

Apply it to blisters of any kind. Use it to shrink warts.

Analgesic

Because it is also a topical analgesic, it will sooth painful shingles eruptions, even around the eyes.

Use it for hemorrhoids and vaginal infections.

Fungicide

Aloe Vera is also a fungicide. And it's better for your feet than antifungal creams. Just apply to the affected area, or put it in a foot bath for a soothing, anti-fungal toenail treatment.

Gastrointestinal Issues

Can You Safely Take Aloe Vera Internally?

The short answer is yes.

The long answer contains cautions. While it is safe to take Aloe Vera gel by the teaspoonful, it is never wise to take it all the time for every condition you may experience. Just like anything, too much is too much.

So how do you use Aloe Vera safely, and what do you use it for? It works well on constipation.

That alone should tell you that too much will cause diarrhea and the health conditions caused by diarrhea, including bloody stools and the inability for the intestines to absorb nutrients and certain medications.

That said, if you have gastrointestinal issues, a small amount, 1 teaspoon, of Aloe Vera taken daily for a few weeks

will not harm you. In fact it may balance out your condition.
If the condition persists or reoccurs, discontinue.

2

Anise

Grow a little Anise in your herb garden. Your

body, and your family, will love you for it.

First of all, you'll need a climate that has hot summers, or your crop will be stunted. Because I live in the mountains, and the summers rarely get above 95 degrees F, and only for a few days. This is not a good climate for Anise. I grew enough for seed to plant, but didn't harvest enough to use for medication. If I wanted Anise for medication, I would need to put my Anise in lots of pots on the railing of my porch where it would get the most sun.

After harvesting, store your seeds in dry, air-tight containers in a dark place. This prevents the essential oils from evaporating.

Benefits of Anise:

Anise seeds (the fruit of the plant) have anti-oxidant, disease preventing properties, in addition to a host of B vitamins, plus vitamins C and A. The seeds also contain minerals like calcium, copper, iron, manganese, magnesium, and potassium. Potassium is an important component in helping to control heart rate and blood pressure.

Anise addresses such problems as:

- Indigestion
- Skin Parasites
- Promoting Mother's Milk
- Coughs, Colds, Congestion and Baby's Colic
- Insomnia

Indigestion

If you have a digestion problem, just chew a few of the seeds after a meal. It also helps with bloating and flatulence. It relieves constipation. Anise has a mild diuretic effect.

Skin Parasites

Apply Anise oil directly to the skin to get rid of parasites, such as lice and scabies. You'll smell good too, a bit like licorice.

Anise Oil

Crush Anise seed just enough to break it apart and release the oils.
Fill bottle almost full with Anise seed.
Pour almond oil into bottle until full, completely submerging the Anise seed.
Cap tightly.
Set on sunny windowsill for about a month, poking a clean knife blade into the oil to release air bubbles every couple of days for the first week.
Strain through cheesecloth into bottle. Cap and store in dark place. Remember to label your bottle so you know what you stored there. I also list what the oil is used for on the bottle.

Anise Tea

1 teaspoon crushed Anise
1 cup boiling water
Pour water into cup with Anise seed.
Let steep 5-20 minutes.

Promoting Mother's Milk

Drink a cup of Anise tea in the evening. Anise Tea promotes your body's ability to make estrogen, so drink daily while needed.

Coughs, Colds, Congestion and Colic
Drink a cup of Anise tea in the evening while symptoms remain. This tea is also gentle enough for baby's colic.

Insomnia
A cup of Anise tea before bed will also help with insomnia.

In Cooking
Use Anise seeds in breads and with meats. Use it in sachets and making your own soaps and lotions.

Anise Extract, for flavoring
Use Star Anise because it has the strongest licorice flavor.

Fill glass jar with whole Anise.

Pour vodka into jar until it reaches the top, cover tightly.

Store in dark, cool place for three months. Shake jar every two weeks.

Taste after three months. If Anise flavor is not strong enough, store for another month or two.

Strain into extract bottle with tight lid. Label and store in cupboard with other extracts.

3

Basil

Basil, a popular herb for chicken and pasta dishes,

is best if used fresh. Its oils weaken as it dries, so to

get enough flavor, you'll need to use more.

The same can be said for using Basil for remedies: the fresher, the better.

Basil has been used for:
- Anti-Inflammatory
- Diabetes
- Respiratory Issues
- Lower Cholesterol
- Toothpaste
- Kidney Stones
- Gastrointestinal Issues
- Eye Drops
- Headaches
- Bug Bites
- Ear Infections

Anti-inflammatory
Basil works is an anti-inflammatory remedy for such conditions as rheumatoid arthritis and bowel inflammations. Drink one cup of Basil Tea slowly.

Basil Tea

1 teaspoon Basil

1 cup boiling water

Pour water into cup with the Basil. Let steep for 10-20 minutes. Drink slowly.

Diabetes

Diabetes is a complicated disease, and drinking Basil Tea, or seasoning food with Basil is only part of the solution. That said, the reason consuming Basil works well for those with diabetes is that it decreases glucose levels while increasing insulin production. It contains cinnamanic acid, which enhanced circulation and stabilizes blood sugar.

Lower Blood Sugar

1 teaspoon Basil leaves

1 cup boiling water.

Pour water over leaves

Let steep 10-20 minutes.

Drink daily to lower blood sugar.

Respiratory Issues

Cinnamanic acid, an active ingredient in Basil, assists the breathing in those with respiratory problems, including allergies. The seeds work to help remove excess mucous, which helps relieve coughs and asthma symptoms. The leaves also have antibiotic properties to treat even drug-resistant infections.

Asthma Tea

Add 1 cup boiling water to 1 teaspoon of Basil with 1/4 teaspoon of ginger. Stir in honey to taste.

To reduce a fever, especially in children, boil 1/2 cup of Basil leaves with a tablespoon of cardamom in 2 quarts of water. Let cool.

Strain and add milk and honey for flavor to each cup served.

Allow fevered child to sip on the liquid throughout the day.

Chewing on Basil leaves, especially fresh Basil (which means you need to grow it inside during the winter), will help with cold and flu symptoms.

Coughs Due to Colds or Flu
Add 1 cup boiling water to 1 teaspoon of Basil, 1/4 teaspoon of cloves, and a pinch of salt. May add honey to taste. Drink this 4 to 5 times a day. You may find that your associated headache will be gone too.

Lower Cholesterol
Daily use of Basil will lower cholesterol and strengthen the heart. Chewing Basil leaves is also good to reduce stress. As a side effect, you may find that bugs don't like to be around you, but people do. One man's comment was, "If all our vegetables tasted like pizza, we would be less likely to refuse them."

Toothpaste
Dried Basil ground to a powder makes a good tooth-cleaning agent to replace toothpaste. In our culture we erroneously believe we need toothpaste in order to clean our teeth. It's the brushing that's important. So your toothbrush is sufficient. But why not add something that can help remedy sore gums and keep gums and the inside of the mouth healthy at the same time? It will make your breath smell fresh too.

Kidney Stones
This has been helpful to eliminate kidney stones through the urine. Chew on fresh Basil leaves daily for 6 months.

Gastrointestinal Issues
1 teaspoon fresh Basil, or 1/2 teaspoon dried
Basil Add 1 cup of boiling water.
Let steep 10 minutes.
Sip slowly.

Eye Drops
Add 1 cup boiling water to 1 teaspoon Basil and let sit for 5 hours at room temperature. Strain liquid into jar. Use 2 drops per eye before bed.

Headache
Add 1 tablespoon dried Basil
To half-filled quart pot of boiling water
Lean over steam
Drape towel over head breathe in steam for 10 minutes

Bug Bites and Stings
Chew some Basil, the apply the chewed Basil to the affected area.

Basil Oil, for Ear Infections Fill jar with fresh Basil.
Add olive oil and let sit in sunny window for 1 month.
Strain oil through cloth, or tea strainer into clean jar.
Store in dark place.
Put 2 drops of oil into affected ear.

4

Bay Leaves

The Bay tree is an evergreen that grows to 30 feet high. But it does not tolerate cold climates, so if you live in a warmer climate, you may want to grow one in your back yard.

Not only does Bay smell and taste good, but it is full of nutrients. Because it is rich in Vitamin B, including folic acid, it is great for pregnant women. The B Vitamins in Bay are good for the nerves. In addition to vitamins, Bay leaves are also rich in minerals such as potassium, calcium, manganese, iron, zinc, and others. These minerals regulate blood pressure, promote healthy blood and help control your heart rate.

Bay has been used for:

- Insect Repellent
- Swollen Joints
- Gastrointestinal Issues
- Sore Throat
- Fever, Pain Relief
- Dandruff
- Insomnia

Insect Repellent
Bay is very handy in the south where mosquitoes are plentiful. Rub some fresh Bay leaves on exposed skin for an insect repellent.

Swollen Joints

Rubbing fresh leaves on swollen joints, sprains and strains has also proven effective.

Gastrointestinal Issues, including colic

To soothe stomach ulcers, digestion complaints, diarrhea, and relieve flatulence, drink a cup of Bay Leaf Tea in the evenings before bed.

Bay Leaf Tea

1 Bay Leaf
1 cup boiling water

Pour water over Bay leaf. Let sit for about 10 minutes.

This tea is mild and can be used for infants with colic.

You can either drink the tea, or add a little salt and use it as a gargle for a sore throat at any time during the day.

Fever Reducer, including pain relief

Bay will ease arthritis and muscle pain, to reduce fever and treat bronchitis and flu symptoms, make a Bay Leaf Tea.

For additional help during the flu season, soak a cloth that has been soaked in boiled Bay leaves and water, and place on the chest as a compress.

Dandruff

Use a Bay Leaf Rinse to reduce dandruff.

Bay Leaf Hair Rinse

1 tablespoon Bay
1 quart boiling water
Put water into jar with Bay Leaf.
Let steep until just warm.
Rinse hair after shampooing.

Insomnia

Because Bay contains a mild narcotic, you can use it to induce sleep. This works well for people with pain, and helps them get a good, healing sleep.

5
BEANS

I know, I know. This isn't an herb. But it is a Power-Food, and your kitchen will not be complete without a variety of Beans.

Beans have been used for:

- Protein
- Blood Sugar
- Cancer Prevention
- Cholesterol
- High Blood Pressure
- Prevent Constipation

Protein

Beans are high in protein. While they are in incomplete protein, meaning they don't have all the necessary amino acids in one package, such as a cut of meat will, the missing amino acids are easy enough to complete with:

- Any Milk Product, such as cheese, milk and yogurt
- Any Grain Product, such as rice and the ingredients for bread or tortillas (wheat and corn)
- Nuts
- Seeds

The exceptions are soy products, such as soy milk and tofu. Soy contains a complete protein.

A note on protein: Humans have different protein requirements from dogs and cats. What makes a complete protein for a human will not suffice for our carnivorous friends. They need meat protein. If they don't get it, they will go blind.

Blood Sugar
Beans help the body regulate blood sugar levels.

Cancer Prevention
Beans also are instrumental in reducing the risk of many cancers.

Cholesterol
Beans are one of the Power-Foods that help to lower cholesterol. Other foods in this category are:

- Fruits, vegetables, especially apples and carrots
- Bananas, grapefruit, oranges, bell peppers, broccoli, spinach
- Onions (raw) and garlic (also raw)
- Nuts, seeds (especially almonds) and whole grains
- Salmon, mackerel, tuna, sardines and other fatty fish
- Oysters and mussels
- Olive oil

High Blood Pressure
Beans lower high blood pressure. Other Power-Foods that lower high blood pressure are:

- Salmon, mackerel, tuna, sardines and other fatty fish
- Fruits and vegetables, especially celery, onions, tomatoes, bananas, spinach and garlic
- Green tea

Prevent Constipation
Beans prevent constipation and regulate the colon. Other Power Foods that prevent constipation are:

- Fresh fruits and vegetables (at least five a day)
- Whole grains

- Water, coffee, tea

Beans should be a part of your weekly diet.

6
Broccoli

This is a Power-Food. When your mother told you to eat your Broccoli, she probably wasn't thinking of preventing cancer. She was probably considering the amazing bounty of vitamins and minerals that broccoli contains. Broccoli is definitely a healthy food. Maybe you mother was thinking of its incredible antioxidant properties.

Broccoli is used for:

- Cancer Prevention
- Lower Cholesterol
- Arthritis Inflammation
- Colds and Allergies (reduces impact)
- Osteoporosis Prevention
- Heart Health
- Detoxifier
- Digestive Aid
- Restless Leg Syndrome
- Increased Brain and Muscle Function
- High Blood Pressure
- Eye Health

Cancer Prevention
Broccoli contains the chemical, indole-3-carbinol, is an anticar-

cinogen. That particular chemical inhibits the growth of breast, cervical and prostate cancers. It also boosts the immune system by strengthening the liver.

Included in this cancer-fighting family are Brussels sprouts, cabbage and cauliflower.

Lower Cholesterol
As a whole food, Broccoli abounds with fiber that pulls cholesterol from your system. This means that it's helpful in reducing cholesterol.

Arthritis Inflammation
Broccoli, with its abundance of omega 3 fatty acids, is an anti-inflammatory food. Do you suffer from painful arthritis flare-ups? Do you have problems with an irritated bowel? Do you have other chronic conditions characterized by inflammation? Eat more Broccoli.

Colds and Allergies
If you have allergies, Broccoli has been known to lessen their impact on your body.

In addition to concentrated amounts of Vitamin C and the flavonoids necessary for Vitamin C to work, Broccoli is a terrific antioxidant. It contains significant amounts of flavonoids such as lutein, zeaxanthin and beta-carotene. So the next time you get a cold, ask yourself: Are you eating enough Broccoli?

Osteoporosis Prevention
Because Broccoli is high in calcium and Vitamin K, it adds to bone health and adds to the prevention of osteoporosis.

Heart Health
Broccoli is part of a heart-healthy diet. Not only will it help your heart stay healthy, and prevent heart disease, there is some evidence that it may actually reverse damage to the linings of your blood vessels caused by chronic high blood sugar levels.

Detoxifier

For a great detoxifier, eat Broccoli. It has chemicals that neutralize and eliminate toxins, even at a genetic level.

Digestive Aid

And because it is part of a low-carb diet and high in fiber, Broccoli aids in your digestion, prevents constipation and helps maintain low blood sugar. Because it is loaded with protein, with half the calories of the same amount of rice or corn, it is the perfect diet food. Plus, because it is an alkaline vegetable, it helps balance your body's acidic levels.

Restless Leg Syndrome

Because Broccoli is high in potassium, it helps maintain a healthy nervous system. Do you suffer from leg cramps, or restless leg syndrome? Eat foods high in potassium. We go to doctors for all kinds of ailments, when eating good food is often the best answer.

Increased Brain and Muscle Function

Broccoli helps maintain a high brain function – all you students pay attention. And all you body builders, Broccoli promotes regular muscle growth.

High Blood Pressure

Do you fight chronic high blood pressure? Broccoli contains high levels of potassium, magnesium and calcium, all of which help regulate your blood pressure.

Eye Health

Are you getting older? You need not lose your eyesight as a result. One ingredient, lutein, can help prevent macular degeneration so prevalent in the elderly, as well as cataracts. The fact that it's also high in Vitamin A is only a plus for continued eye health.

Further Note on Eating

Although we, in the United States, have been known in the past as the most well-fed nation on the planet, we have one huge defect. We don't know how to eat. Oh, we know how to diet, but not how to eat. Even though birth defects are not common, one or two babies per 1,000 are born with a cleft palate or a spinal cord defect. The cause is that the mother did not get enough folate during pregnancy. Although the cause for these defects can also be because the infant's body, for whatever reason, cannot absorb enough folate, it need not be because the mother isn't getting enough. Doctors prescribe prenatal vitamins to help correct this problem. But you can correct it yourself with a diet full of this nutrient.

Broccoli is not hard to grow. Indeed, you can even grow it inside your apartment if you don't have any land. Do not cut your nutrition to save a dollar. Make sure your food money goes to feed you.

7

Caraway

Caraway is an herb that is great in salads, especially fruit salads, in breads, especially rye breads, in cakes, and in baked fruit desserts, especially baked apple desserts.

As a Medicine
The parts of the caraway that can be used are the seeds, leaves and roots. Dry them first before using.

Caraway can be used for:

- Detoxifier
- Stomach Disorders
- Bad Breath
- Earache
- Bruises

Detoxifier
Caraway is a natural detoxifier. It increases kidney action, and can relieve flatulence. It also can be used with other medicines to reduce nausea and stomach cramps.

Stomach Disorders
For colic, to counter the adverse effects of some medicines, to reduce flatulence, you can make a tea that can be taken three times a day.

Caraway Tea
To make a caraway tea, boil 1 teaspoon of seeds in 1-2 liters of water for 15 minutes.
Strain.

May be served either hot or warm. Please only serve it warm for babies with colic, unless you want a screaming infant on your hands.

Bad Breath
Chew a few caraway seeds to take away bad breath, or a bad taste in the mouth.

Earache
Mash Caraway seeds and place in a hot cloth. Hold cloth to the affected ear.

Bruises
Pound Caraway seeds into a paste to help heal bruises.

NOTE of CAUTION: Although Caraway works for indigestion in small amounts, too much can cause heartburn. Caraway oil must also be used judiciously. Taken over too long a time can cause liver and kidney damage. Caraway must NOT be taken by pregnant women. It may cause abortion. Caraway may have a mild narcotic effect, causing drowsiness and nausea.

8
Carrots

Carrots are a Power Food. Your mother always told you

to eat your vegetables. What she probably didn't tell

you was to eat them raw. But raw Carrots are best.

Carrots are not difficult to grow in your garden. I live in a trailer park, so the land is not mine, but I have half-barrels that I use for my herbs and gardens, plus a variety of pots. Carrots grow well in pots. You need good soil that has plenty of room for their roots. Or you can grow shorter varieties, which are more ideal for patio plants.

You can also grow them in your house in pots during the winter. Why depend on the grocery store, if you have a sunny window?

Carrots have been used for:

- Improving Vision
- Cancer Prevention
- Anti-Aging
- Beautiful Skin
- Acne
- Detoxifier and Heart Health
- Tooth Decay Prevention

Improving Vision
Carrots really do improve your vision, especially your night vi-

sion. But what you might not know is that Carrots also help prevent macular degeneration as well as cataracts. See better. Eat a carrot a day.

Cancer Prevention

What you may not know, however, is that carrots also prevent cancer. Carrots contain falcarinol and falcarindiol. Now, that means nothing to me, but researchers have recently found that these are anti-cancer properties. Wouldn't you like anti-cancer properties swimming around in your system?

Anti-Aging

There are also anti-aging properties in Carrots. Good to know! Although we can't prevent old age, we can prevent some of the wear and tear life gives us.

One of the benefits of anti-aging properties is that you can maintain that vibrant, glowing skin look. Carrots prevent premature wrinkles, acne, dry skin, in addition to an uneven skin tone. Look youthful. Eat a Carrot!

Beautiful Skin

Do you want beautiful skin? Try a Carrot facial mask. Just steam a Carrot until it's soft, add a teaspoon of honey, a teaspoon of olive oil, and a few drops of lemon, and mash together. Put on your face for up to 10 minutes, then wash off, and pat your face dry. Be beautiful. Enjoy a Carrot facial!

Acne

Cuts or acne, cooked or raw, Carrots can also be used to treat skin infections and cuts.

Detoxifier and Heart Health

Do yourself an additional favor. As the Carrots you are now eating cleans toxins from your body, you can lower your cholesterol while you also prevent heart disease. A dynamic duo of healthy benefits! And just think how you're cleaning out the rest of your body. As you lower cholesterol and save your heart, you are also cleaning out your colon.

Did I mention that as you lower cholesterol you are also preventing a stroke? Has your doctor told you that you are a health risk for certain conditions? Stroke need not be one of them.

Tooth Decay Prevention

And, as you munch on your new-found health food, you'll also be cleaning your teeth and gums. Carrots help eliminate plaque and prevent tooth decay.

Say hello to your new best friend—your Carrot!

9

Cayenne

The active ingredient in Cayenne is capsaicin. That's what's responsible for the heat you feel in your hands when you forget to put on gloves when you cut them up, or that heat you feel in your throat when you pepper your food with Cayenne. It's a natural heat, and it works very well for some things.

Cayenne has been used for:

- Muscle Aches and Nerve Pain
- Circulation
- Digestive Problems
- Headaches
- Toothaches, Mouthwash
- Sprains
- Colds and Infections
- Fatigue
- Cuts and Scrapes
- Chest Congestion

Muscle Aches and Nerve Pain
Cayenne has been used for centuries for muscle ache and nerve pain, such as sore muscles due to strenuous exercise or the pain of arthritis and bursitis.

Circulation

Cayenne can help restore circulation. To keep your feet warm and the blood circulating in the winter, sprinkle some Cayenne powder into your shoes or boots. It has also been used in frostbite cases.

Digestive Problems
If you like the taste of Cayenne, you can sprinkle some on your food to help with digestive problems.

If you don't want Cayenne flavoring your meal, you can also add 1/8th teaspoon of Cayenne powder into a glass of water for indigestion or stomach problems. This also works for constipation.

Headaches
Cayenne works on headaches too. Just rub a little Cayenne Cream on your temples. If the headache is from sinuses, you can make a nasal spray with a pinch of Cayenne into enough water to fill a nasal spray bottle. Shake well before using.

For a hangover, drink 1/8th teaspoon of Cayenne powder in a glass of water.

Toothaches
To relieve a toothache, you can use Cayenne oil on a piece of cotton and swab the tooth and gums with the cloth.

Mouthwash
Cayenne can also be used as a mouthwash. 1/8th teaspoon in a glass of water works as a mouthwash.

Sprains
Painful sprain? Make a Cayenne liniment rub by boiling a tablespoon of Cayenne powder in a pint of apple cider vinegar, and apply some with a cloth to the sprain. You will want to use gloves before applying.

Colds and Infections
Cayenne also fights colds and infections. Cayenne is loaded with

Vitamin C. It's good for sore throats, laryngitis and coughs too. Add 1/8th of a teaspoon of Cayenne powder to a glass of warm water. Stir and drink, or gargle for laryngitis.

Fatigue
Combine Cayenne powder with Ginseng to fight fatigue. Both are also good for your heart.

Cuts and Scrapes
For minor bleeding, just sprinkle Cayenne powder right on the scrape or cut. It works wonders.

Chest Congestion
As a poultice or liniment, Cayenne works well for chest congestion.

Making Cayenne Medicinal Topicals

Note the difference between a liniment and a poultice: A liniment is the liquid applied to the affected area with a cloth. A poultice is a cloth saturated in the liquid or a paste applied directly to the affected area.

Medicinal Drink, for Colds, Coughs, Sore Throats, Digestive Complaints
1/8th teaspoon to 1 cup water
Mix well and drink (or gargle if for laryngitis)
Works as a mouthwash too.

Cayenne Liniment, for Arthritis and Sprains
1 tablespoon Cayenne powder to 1 pint of apple cider vinegar.
Boil gently for about 10 minutes.
Do not strain. Pour liquid into a jar and use as needed.
For external use only.

Poultice or Compress, for Chest Congestion, Sprains, Arthritis, Sore Joints and Muscles

1 tablespoon Cayenne powder to 1 pint of apple cider vinegar. Boil gently for about 10 minutes.

Cool slightly, but keep remaining mixture warm. You will want to keep changing the cloths to warm compresses as they cool.

Dip clean cloth in mixture and apply directly to affected area. Leave compress on affected area. Change cloth to warm cloth as it cools.

Cayenne Oil, for Massage, Arthritis, Sore Joints and Muscles
1/2 teaspoon Cayenne powder to 1 cup warm olive oil or grape-seed oil.
Mix well.
Apply to sore, aching muscles and joints. Massage in.

Cayenne Cream, for sore muscles and joints
2 tablespoons Cayenne powder
2 cups olive or sunflower oil
Heat together on low heat for about 2 hours.
Strain mixture through a clean cloth or tea strainer (my favorite)
Add 1 ½ ounces of beeswax and stir on low heat until beeswax is melted.
Pour mixture into airtight container and allow it to thicken into a cream.
Apply to affected area as needed for pain.

10
Chives

Chives are a multi-purpose plant. The whole plant can be used, the bulbs, the leaves, stems and flowers. For maximum benefit as a medicine, Chives are best when fresh, but dried Chives still can be added to soups, salads, and other foods.

To keep Chives available year around, keep a pot of them growing in your kitchen. Chives make an excellent part of a kitchen herbal garden.

Chives have been used for:

- Antibacterial Agent
- Hearth Health
- Digestive Aid
- Cancer
- Garden Aid

Antibacterial Agent

Crush the leaves and bulbs into a paste and apply them directly to cuts, bites and wounds.

Heart Health

This member of the onion family is rich in flavonoids that help to stabilize and reduce blood pressure, and lower cholesterol. Because it is high in Vitamin C, Chives help keep the walls of the capillaries flexible and help the body to absorb iron. Your only problem when using Chives is to get enough of them. You may consider using them more often in various foods, or making them a regular part of your vegetable and herb intake.

Digestive Aid
Because Chives are high in fiber, they are good for your digestion, and contribute to the health of your intestines. Chives can prevent constipation and hemorrhoids. But eating too many at any one time can irritate the stomach.

Cancer
Not only does eating Chives regularly resist cancer, it actually inhibits the growth of tumors. It is helpful in treating esophageal, stomach, prostate and gastrointestinal tract cancers.

Chive Tea Uses
There are three ways to use Chive teas. In the mild form, it has been used to treat diarrhea, to get rid of gas, to help cough up mucous, to strengthen the heart, and as part of a spring tonic. In the stronger form it has been used as a mild analgesic, an antiseptic and a topical disinfectant. In a very strong form it has even been use as a fungicide and bacterial infections.

A very mild tea may be given to pregnant women to help increase their nutrition and the health of their unborn infants.
Eating Chives and other members of the onion family reduces the rate of getting prostate cancer.
Chives are also a part of a heart-healthy diet. By eating Chives regularly, you lower you high cholesterol levels. It has been used to lower high blood pressure.

So if the only times you eat Chives is on your baked potato, you might want to consider other ways to incorporate Chives into your diet. Think of salads, soup and stews, in breads, on top of chili, in pasta dishes, and even in a daily tea.

Chive Tea:

Start with 1 teaspoon of chopped Chive tops to one cup of boiling water. Let steep for 10 minutes.

If this is too strong, add more water.

For stronger teas, you may add more Chives, steep longer, or both.

You will need to experiment with the strength, depending on the purpose of your remedy.

Garden Aid

Do you have a mole problem in your garden? Plant more Chives. The juice can even be used as a moth repellent, as well as an insect repellent.

How To Grow Chives

Method One – In A Cold Frame:

Early in the spring, start your seeds inside a cold frame. When the seedlings are large enough to handle, ease them out of the cold frame and put three to a pot. Then plant the Chive clumps in their permanent location. The following spring, you can divide larger clumps into smaller clumps and thereby extend your Chive garden or border.

Method Two – Inside Your Home

Start the seeds inside a tray. Keep moist. When the seedlings are large enough to handle, put them in their permanent pots in a sunny window.

11

Cinnamon

I almost didn't put this common spice into this book, because cinnamon is so expensive. Also, there is a debate as to whether cassia is true cinnamon. It is, it's just not Ceylon cinnamon, which is very expensive. So most stores now sell cassia instead of the cinnamon from Celon. They taste the same.

Cinnamon has been used for:

- Cholesterol
- Blood Sugar
- Yeast Infection
- Cancer Prevention
- Anti-Clotting
- Arthritis
- Antibacterial
- Brain Health
- E-Coli

Cholesterol

In recent studies, a mere smidgen, no more than 1/2 teaspoon of Cinnamon will lower LDL cholesterol levels.

Perhaps you'd like some Cinnamon in your next cup of coffee or tea. It could help.

Blood Sugar

In another study, there was evidence that Cinnamon may actually regulate the blood sugar in people with Type II Diabetes. If you are diabetic or pre-diabetic, give this some thought. That extra bit of Cinnamon on your next dessert might be healthy for you.

Yeast Infections
Not all yeast infections respond to medication. Should that be the case with you, try an extra 1/2 teaspoon daily of Cinnamon could be amazingly beneficial.

Cancer Prevention
Although it may not work once cancer has a firm hold on you, Cinnamon has been shown reduce the spread of lymphoma and leukemia cancer cells.

Anti-Clotting
If your blood has a tendency to clot easily, or if you need your blood to be a bit thinner, consider adding 1/2 teaspoon of Cinnamon to your diet each day.

Arthritis
Arthritis is an auto-immune disease, meaning, the body attacks itself as if it were a germ. There are many arthritis remedies available both with and without prescriptions. All of those drugs relieve the pain, but they cause other damage to your body.

In a recent study, 1/2 teaspoon of cinnamon was added to 1 teaspoon of honey and taken before breakfast every morning. Arthritis sufferers reported a significant decrease in pain after only one week. After a month, those people could walk without pain.

The best news? Their bodies didn't have to also fight the side effects of manufactured arthritis drugs as well.

Antibacterial
Cinnamon has been shown to slow down bacterial growth in foods to which it has been added. It is a *natural* food preservative. That's why our grandparents were safe when they left desserts with Cinnamon added to them, such as your apple and

pumpkins pies, on the counter for the next day's feast, without refrigeration.

Now, if you're going to leave your desserts out for a week, you might need to rethink that. Nothing works as a preservative forever.

Brain Health

Ready for something amazing? One study discovered that just the act of *smelling* Cinnamon increased mental acuity.

E-Coli

Want to keep your juices safe a little longer? Cinnamon added to unpasteurized juices fights the presence of the E. coli bacteria. Keep a little Cinnamon on hand, if only for that.

Risks

Please be aware that taken in high quantities of the cassia form of Cinnamon may prove toxic.

Also, those with hormone-sensitive cancers, such as breast cancer should not take Cinnamon.

Diabetics taking Cinnamon should be aware that they may need to adjust their medication after taking it for a while.

12

Cinnamon and Honey

Honey and Cinnamon together make a dynamic duo. Honey has antiseptic and antibacterial agents. Combined with Cinnamon's properties, you have a winning combination.

Honey and Cinnamon have been used for:

- Heart Health
- Arthritis
- Bladder Infections
- Cholesterol
- Colds
- Immune System Booster
- Gastrointestinal Issues
- Insect Bites

Heart Health

Do you like peanut butter and jelly sandwiches? Do you like a little jelly on your toast? For a healthier heart and to dissolve the plaque that causes hardening of the arteries and strokes, substitute a spread made with Honey and Cinnamon.

Arthritis

The above spread is also good if you have arthritis. But you could also increase the benefit of this duo by making an Arthritis Tea.

Arthritis Tea

1 cup hot water
2 teaspoons Honey

1 teaspoon Cinnamon
Mix together and drink three times a day to ease arthritis pain.

Bladder Infections
Who gets bladder infections? Newlyweds do. This isn't talked about very often, but because of the frequency of sex, sometimes bacteria gets pushed into the urethra causing a bladder infection. So do those who don 't drink enough water. Dehydration causes the bladder to be unable to eliminate toxins effectively, making bladder infections more likely.

Bladder Infection Tea
1 cup warm water
2 tablespoons Cinnamon
1 teaspoon Honey
Mix together
Drink once per day until urine runs clear.

Cholesterol
Not everyone develops high cholesterol as they get older, and a person doesn't need to be overweight to get this condition either. But for those who do, add 2 tablespoons of Honey and 3 tablespoons of Cinnamon to your tea once a day.

Colds
Everyone gets them. It's time to know what to do when you do. At the first sign of a cold, take one teaspoon of Honey laced with 1/4 teaspoon of Cinnamon for three days in a row. This helps clear sinuses and reduce coughing.

Immune System Booster
Cinnamon and Honey together, no matter which recipe you use, strengthens the immune system. Put it in your hot cereal, on your toast, use both instead of plain sugar. Stay healthy.

Gastrointestinal Issues

Sprinkle a little Cinnamon over a teaspoon of honey before meals to reduce stomach complaints.

13

Cloves

The purpose of food is to feed you and give you more than just enough fuel for the day. Food's job is to saturate your body in healthy nutrition. The problem with junk food is that it doesn't feed you. It robs your body of nutrition so that your body, just in order to digest the junk food, has to remove health from your body just to get the junk processed.

Cloves fall into the category of a Super Spice. In other words, of all the spices in your cupboard, Cloves tops the list. It has more antioxidants, more antiseptic, more germicidal, and more antiinflammatory properties than all the rest. In fact, of all the foods in your kitchen, cloves have the highest antioxidant value of any food!

Cloves have been used for:
- Anti-Inflammation
- Analgesic
- Antiseptic and Germacide
- Gastrointestinal Issues
- Immune System Booster
- Mental Acuity
- High Blood Pressure

Anti-Inflammation
Cloves fight inflammation, such as the inflammation of arthritis and other conditions.

Analgesic
One of the most well-known uses for Cloves is to stop the pain of toothaches. A little oil of Clove on a cotton swab applied to the tooth works wonders. Or soak a cotton ball in oil of Clove and apply to sore gums as well as the infected tooth for even more relief.

Cloves are very potent. You may decide that a whole cotton ball soaked in Clove oil is too much. You can take some ground Cloves and wrap in a small cloth or patch of coffee filter and place on the affected area just as effective.

Cloves will also draw out infection, so it will prevent the tooth from abscessing. You can then see the dentist without having to go on antibiotics first.

Antiseptic and Germicide
Cloves, having antiseptic and germicide properties, work against any infection, including colds, flu and other respiratory issues. For coughs and colds, put either oil of clove or a tablespoon of clove powder into a pot of boiling water. Remove the pot from the fire and put a towel over your head and breathe in the steam for about 10 minutes.

Mental Acuity
Because regular use of Cloves is beneficial to blood circulation, and because oxygenated blood is vital to memory and brain function, Cloves is an idea spice to add daily to your diet.

High Blood Pressure
Drink some Clove Tea daily, and chew on a whole clove every so often. This will help reduce high blood pressure.

Clove Pomander

A Clove Pomander has multiple uses. It will aid in respiration, freshen the air and deter flies for about six months.

To make the Clove Pomander, take a fresh orange and insert whole Cloves randomly over the surface of the orange. Tie a string or ribbon around the orange and hang wherever you and your family are most likely to congregate.

14

Coffee

Coffee is many people's favorite drink. The smell of a freshly brewed cup, a morning sun brightening the window, the day's troubles still a bit into the future, these moments of time before the rush are to be cherished.

Coffee is a stimulant. It stimulates awareness and concentration, elevates mood, and quickens responses. The coffee's chemicals don't quite dissipate for four to six hours after that final cup. Some people find that it will keep them awake too long, but everyone's body is different. Some find that coffee puts them right to sleep, and some never like the edgy feeling that it can give them.

Coffee helps in several ways:

- Mental Acuity
- Heart Health
- Diabetes
- Diminished Pain
- Weight Loss
- Lower Risk of Death
- Reduce Risk of Cancer

Mental Acuity
Although Alzheimer's is a complicated disease, recent studies have shown that three to five cups of coffee daily delayed the

onset. In sixty-five percent of the cases, it decreased the chances of developing Alzheimer's entirely.

Heart Health
Studies are still going on, but a single cup of coffee daily has been shown to reduce the risk of cardiovascular disease death by as much as thirty-eight percent.

Diabetes
Type II diabetes is another complicated disease. One Harvard study found that those who drank coffee had a reduced risk of developing the disease. Drinking coffee is no guarantee, of course, but the risk of the onset of type II diabetes was significantly reduced in the study.

Analgesic
Many people suffer pain throughout the day. Those who took an afternoon coffee break, in one Norwegian study, dealt with less pain. So if you're having a difficult day, drink a cup of coffee. It could help.

Weight Loss
One study proved people taking a green coffee extract lost weight. By itself, drinking a nicely brewed cup of coffee has not proved to help people lose weight. But you might look into a green coffee extract if you're having issues with weight.

Lower Risk of Death
Regardless of whether a person drank decaffeinated or caffeinated coffee, studies have shown that those who drank three cups of coffee daily, or more, lowered their risk of death from several causes, specifically heart disease and diabetes.

Reduce Risk of Cancer
Lower risk of prostate cancer, endometrial cancer, skin cancer and oral cancer are some of the cancers that studies have found to reduce risks in getting.

So the next time someone wants to ask if you'd like another cup of coffee, just say, "Yes, I think I will." And never feel guilty again for liking that next cup.

15

Cilantro

Cilantro is the herb. Coriander is the seed. This herb is used in so many foods, it's almost a necessity around here (southwestern United States).

When I researched other uses for Cilantro, I was pleased to discover that it has been used as a remedy for quite a few conditions:

- Gastrointestinal Issues
- Diarrhea
- Diuretic
- Cholesterol
- Topical Pain Reliever
- Skin Problems
- Antihistamine
- Salmonella Protection
- Anemia
- Bone Health
- Viruses
- Menstrual Disorders
- Eye Care
- Blood Sugar
- Cancer

Gastrointestinal Issues

Chew on a few seeds, or drink a tea made from the seeds.

Diarrhea

Cilantro also helps regulate the bowels and clean the liver. If the diarrhea is due to a fungal or microbial infection, drinking Strong Cilantro Tea slowly until symptoms ease will work.

Diuretic
Drink one cup of Cilantro Tea daily for a diuretic effect.

Mild Cilantro Tea
1 cup boiling water
1 teaspoon Cilantro leaves and seeds
Pour water over seeds and let steep 10-20 minutes.
Sip slowly.

Strong Cilantro Tea
1 tablespoon Cilantro leaves and seeds
2 to 4 cups boiling water
Boil together for five minutes. Let steep for 5-14 minutes longer.
Strain.
Sip slowly.

A stronger tea can be made for a topical antiseptic, on eczema, or as an antifungal.

Use a stronger tea for curing diarrhea caused by microbes and fungal infections.

High Cholesterol
Eating fresh Cilantro leaves, such as in salsa and on food can be instrumental in elevating the levels of HDL ("good" cholesterol).

Mouth Ulcers
Add a little salt to Cilantro Tea and gargle twice a day.

Topical Pain Reliever, for rheumatism and other topical pain relief
1 teaspoon Coriander seeds
1/2 cup water
Oatmeal to make desired consistency

Apply to affected area

Skin Inflammation, Antifungal, Eczema
Instead of drinking Cilantro Tea, apply it to affected area, or make a Topical Pain Reliever paste (see above) and apply to affected area.

Antihistamine
Unless you are allergic to Cilantro a tea made with either leaves or seeds have an antihistamine effect.

Salmonella Protection
Cilantro contains high levels of dodecenal, a natural antibiotic that counteracts deadly salmonella food poisoning. So if you suspect the food being served, eat some salsa with Cilantro in it. If you're already sick from food poisoning, sip some Mild Cilantro Tea.

Anemia
Because Cilantro is high in iron, it helps correct low iron-caused anemia. Some of the symptoms of low iron anemia are shortness of breath, heart palpitations and extreme fatigue.

Bone Health
Cilantro leaves are also high in calcium. You could enjoy salsa daily!
Yumm!

Viruses (including Smallpox)
Because Cilantro contain anti-bacterial, anti-oxidant, anti-infection and detoxifying properties, and because the leaves are high in Vitamin C, this is an all-purpose ailment for a variety of conditions.

Menstrual Disorders
Cilantro regulates secretions from the endocrine glands, and regulates hormones. As a result, it can regulate periods, and even reduce the associated pain.

Eye Care

Cilantro is full of antioxidants, Vitamin A, Vitamin C, and a variety of minerals that keep eyes healthy and treat conjunctivitis. Make a tea using both seeds and leaves for maximum effect. You can also use this tea to prevent and minimize the effects of macular degeneration, a degrading of vision in the elderly.

Blood Sugar

Drink a Cilantro Tea daily to regulate blood sugar levels.

Cancer

Cilantro-based salsa or tea helps prevent colon cancer.

16

Dill

Everyone who does home canning knows the value of dill sprigs to make a batch of pickles or dilly beans (dilled fresh green beans). But those lovely dill heads, as well as the leaves and seeds, can be used for so much more.

DO NOT USE DILL IF ALREADY PREGNANT

Dill has been used for:

- Digestive Disorders
- Breath Freshener
- Insomnia
- Osteoporosis
- Diabetes
- Arthritis
- Immune System
- Diarrhea
- Menstruation

Digestive Disorders
Drink a cup of Dill Tea slowly for digestive disorders.

Mild Dill Tea
1   teaspoon Dill seeds (crushed)
1 cup boiling water
Pour water over crushed seeds
Let steep for 10 to 15 minutes

Strain
Add honey for sweetening
May drink up to twice a day

Strong Dill Tea
1teaspoons Dill seeds (crushed)
1 cup boiling water
Pour water over crushed seeds.
Let steep 20 minutes.
Strain.
Add honey for sweetening. May drink up to twice a day

.

Breath Freshener
Chew a few Dill seeds as a breath freshener. It also works as a germicide to help keep the mouth healthy.

Insomnia
Drink a cooled cup of Dill Tea an hour before bed.

Fight Osteoporosis, and help mend broken bones
Dill leaves, heads and seeds are high in calcium.
Use the Strong Dill Tea twice a day to help fight Osteoporosis and to help mend broken bones

Diabetes
Dill Tea and Dill seeds help regulate insulin levels.

Arthritis
Dill is an anti-inflammatory. It helps reduce the inflammation and pain of arthritis, gout, and rheumatoid arthritis.

Immune System
Dill helps strengthen the immune system because it is an anti-micro biotic. This anti-microbial activity helps the system fight infections of all kinds, from those things that would cause infections, such as wounds and cuts.

Diarrhea

There are two things that can cause chronic diarrhea: parasites and microbes. As mentioned above, Dill helps with indigestion caused by an unfriendly microbe. And the same ingredients that strengthen the immune system, its anti-microbial agent helps treat the second cause.

This same agent, which is an antioxidant, also helps prevent and fight cancer.

Menstruation

Dill helps the body secrete certain hormones that help the woman's body maintain a balanced menstrual cycle. It's because of the secretion of this hormone that it is wise for women who are already pregnant to NOT use Dill. If a pregnant woman suffers from indigestion, she should use another remedy for her nausea.

17

Fennel

If you plan to grow Fennel in your garden, you will

find that its flower heads looks very much like Dill,

lovely umbrellas of tiny yellow flowers.

Fennel is a fine complement to fish dishes. Just sprinkle some hand-crushed (or mortar-and-pestle crushed) seeds over the fish, either before or after cooking.

You can also take some crushed seeds as an addition to cheese spreads. It's tasty on vegetables, in soups, and as a spice. Many love Fennel as an addition to curry sauces, or chew it after eating a rich meal to aid digestion. Delicious!

For medicinal purposes, all parts of the plant may be used.

Fennel has been used for:

> • Breath Freshener
> • Digestive Aid
> • Constipation and Diarrhea
> • Clean a Sick Room
> • Kidney Stones
> • Weight Loss
> • Anemia
> • Menopause, PMS, Menstrual Disorders
> • Respiratory Ailments

- Immune System
- Heart Disease
- Cancer
- Eye Care
- Blood Pressure
- Brain Function
- Fleas
- Facial

Breath Freshener
Either chew a handful of Fennel seeds, or gargle a tea made with crushed Fennel.

Fennel Tea:
1 teaspoon Fennel seeds
1 cup boiling water
Pour water over crushed seeds. Let steep for 10-15 minutes. Sip slowly.

Fennel Tea helps to settle a too-rich meal, settle indigestion, and cures flatulence. It is common practice in some parts of the world to chew a few seeds after each meal to aid in digestion and freshen the breath.

If there are foods your body has trouble digesting, such as cabbage or beans, chewing a few seeds after a meal will help. The stalks can be eaten like celery.

Constipation and Diarrhea
Does this sound confusing, for something to treat both conditions? Let me put it this way: both are related to the digestion.

One of the main causes of constipation is not drinking enough water, or eating too-salty foods, or foods that don't have anything in them to move the bowels, such as foods made with white flour. Fennel seeds help correct this problem because they have natural fiber.

Diarrhea can be caused by too much sugar in the diet, an improper and non-nutritious diet, and unfriendly bacteria in the intestines. In this case, because Fennel is a natural antibiotic, drinking Fennel teal will help solve this problem.

Also, the bulb of the Fennel is high in Vitamin C, and is a very effective anti-bacterial agent, so it will help with diarrhea associated with the flu.

Clean a Sick Room
To clean the sickroom, boil the leaves, and wash all surfaces with Fennel water.

Kidney Stones
The tea taken 2-3 times a day can help break up kidney stones, making them easier to pass in the urine.

Weight Loss
Fennel tea taken during the hour before a meal can curb your appetite, and thus becomes an aid to weight loss.

Or, you can chew a teaspoon of crushed seeds during the hour before the meal for the same result.

Anemia
In addition to iron, with which hemoglobin is made, Fennel also contains histidine, an amino acid that stimulates the production of hemoglobin. So if your anemia is caused by iron-poor blood, Fennel will address the problem

Menopause, Menstrual Disorders, PMS. Increase Mother's Milk
Fennel seeds and Fennel tea have been used for thousands of years to increase lactation. Some have even claimed it increases breast size.

However, a topical paste can be made to relieve breast swelling, common in the first few weeks of nursing.

It also helps regulate menstrual periods, and its mild analgesic properties can ease painful periods

Some of the symptoms associated with PMS and menopause can also be addressed with Fennel tea because it helps balance hormones.

Respiratory Ailments
Fennel tea with honey makes an excellent tea for coughs and bronchitis because it has expectorant qualities. Crush dried Fennel leaves into a powder and place in a gelatin capsule when drinking a tea is not available. The properties in Fennel help to break up congestion and phlegm, and work to cleanse the body of the toxins that cause respiratory ailments.

Immune System
For the immune system you use the Fennel bulb which is rich in antioxidants and Vitamin C. Vitamin C is instrumental in overall system health, it helps form collagen, produces and repairs skin tissue and protects blood vessel walls. Its antioxidant properties protect the cells from the harmful effects free radicals. The Fennel bulb, as an overall system conditioner, removes blockages in the intestines and flushes harmful toxins out of the system.

Heart Disease
Because of its antioxidant properties, all parts of Fennel are great for heart health. Fennel is an excellent source of fiber, which is why it's so good for digestion and helps reduce unhealthy levels of cholesterol in the blood. These two factors, the elimination of high levels of LDL cholesterol and antioxidant properties, reduce the chances of heart disease, atherosclerosis and strokes.

Cancer
Actual studies have been done on Fennel seed extract as successful in protecting a person from cancer (specifically prostate cancer) and from keeping a person healthy during radiation and chemo cancer treatments. It has been shown to inhibit the

growth of tumors.

The best protection from cancer is to prevent it in the first place. When polio was rampaging through this country, there were whole communities that had either no, or very few cases of this deadly virus. The key ingredient that prevented the virus from taking hold in EVERY case was good nutrition. This is the same with cancer.

Eat well and NEVER DELIBERATLY EXPOSE YOURSELF TO CARCINOGENS.

Eye Care
Fennel protects against inflammation. A weak fennel tea, thoroughly strained, can be used as an eye wash for treating conjunctivitis in infected eyes. In addition, fresh Fennel leaves can be made into a cold compress to be applied over the eyes to reduce irritation and eye fatigue. Its overall health properties in keeping skin cells, blood wall cells and others, also keep eye tissue healthy.

Blood Pressure
To lower blood pressure you need a diet rich in potassium. Potassium relaxes the tension of blood vessels. And one reason to lower salt intake is that diets NOT rich in potassium cannot process excessive salt. Fennel is a great source of potassium.

1 cup of Fennel bulb daily will solve your high blood pressure issues.

Brain Function
Potassium, as just mentioned, also increases brain function. It increases electrical conduction throughout the body, and the body to the brain. It also increases the amount of oxygen that reaches the brain, which increases brain function and cognitive quality.

Fleas

Fleas don't like Fennel. Apply crushed Fennel around bedding and in doorways for a pleasant deodorizer as well as to repel fleas.

Facial

While steeping your Fennel Tea, bend over the steam, with a cloth tented around you, and breathe in the steam. It will open your pores and rejuvenate your facial skin.

NOTE: Do not overuse Fennel. This is not a tea you can drink by the quart. Too much can cause adverse effects.

18
Garlic

Every herb, backyard and indoor garden needs garlic. It is one of the most important herbs you can grow. Furthermore, it is one of the safest you can use, with scientifically proven medicinal properties.

Fresh garlic is best for medicinal uses. Once you cook it, you destroy its medicinal effectiveness. Although cooked garlic still tastes good.

Garlic has been used for:

- Antibacterial
- Antiviral
- Cuts, Wounds, Abrasions
- High Blood Pressure
- Earaches
- Toothaches
- Respiratory Ailments
- Sore Throat

Anti-Bacterial

Garlic is an excellent anti-bacterial agent. You can apply crushed Garlic directly to an open cut, or you can dress a wound with Garlic Oil before binding.

Garlic Oil (for topical use, such as wounds, skin irritations, even athlete's foot and other fungus infections):

1/2 cup fresh, sliced Garlic cloves
Fill jar with cut or smashed Garlic cloves.
Pour olive oil into jar until all garlic cloves are covered. Let the mixture sit on your sunny windowsill for 4-6 weeks.

Strain into bottle with a lid that closes tightly, label and store in a dark place.

Anti-Viral

Garlic helps the body internally. It not only is an anti-bacterial agent, it also has anti-viral properties. To make a tincture for taking Garlic internally, make a Garlic Tincture.

Garlic Tincture (for internal problems):
Soak 1/4 pound of peeled, separated garlic cloves in 1/2 quart of brandy.
Seal tightly.
Shake daily for 2 weeks.
Strain and bottle remainder.
Take in drops, up to 30 drops daily, if needed.

High Blood Pressure, also heart disease, high cholesterol, prevent blood clots.
Take 1-2 chopped cloves of fresh Garlic daily.

Earaches
Put 1-2 drops if Garlic Oil in affected ear.

Toothaches
Put 2-4 drops of Garlic Oil on affected tooth.

Respiratory Ailments, due to coughs or colds
If you are suffering with a chronic cough or have come down with a cold, you can use Garlic Syrup.

Garlic Syrup (for respiratory ailments):
Slice 1 pound of fresh garlic.
Pour 1 quart of boiling water over sliced garlic.
Let sit for 12 hours.
Stir in sugar or honey until the consistency of cough syrup.

Garlic Tea (for sore throat)
Steep several cloves of Garlic in 1/2 cup of water overnight. In morning, hold nose to drink it, unless the smell doesn't bother you.
Let cool, then strain into bottle and cap tightly.

Store Garlic in dark, cool, dry place with good circulation.

19

Ginger

If you have a chronic inflammatory disease, such as diverticulitis, arthritis, gallbladder inflammation, and heart disease, please note that Ginger is the remedy for you. Ginger blocks the enzymes that contribute to the problem, better than anti-inflammatory drugs either over the counter or by prescription.

Furthermore, Ginger doesn't irritate your stomach like many of those drugs do. So if you want a safe, effective remedy for the chronic pain of inflammatory diseases, take a closer look at Ginger.

Ginger has been used for:

- Ovarian Cancer Treatment
- Colon Cancer Prevention
- Morning Sickness and Motion Sickness
- Inflammatory Diseases
- Heartburn
- Migraine
- Colds and Flu
- Menstrual Cramps
- Prevention of Diabetic Neuropathy

Ovarian Cancer
In one study, Ginger actually killed ovarian cancer cells. So if you

have ovarian cancer, feel free to enjoy Ginger liberally.

Colon Cancer

In addition, in another study, Ginger slowed the growth of color-ectal cancer.

Morning Sickness and Motion Sickness

Many doctors prescribe Vitamin B6 for morning sickness. It has been shown that Ginger can provide the same relief, although there is nothing wrong with taking Vitamin B6. It worked well for motion sickness also.

Inflammatory Diseases

A study has shown that Ginger works well to reduce inflammation in diseases such as arthritis. The key is to drink Ginger Tea before each meal.

Ginger Tea

Caution: Ginger is sensitive to both heat and light, so do not overheat this tea. And do not store remaining Ginger in the refrigerator. Store it in a dark cupboard. Use within 3 weeks.

Cut a two-inch piece of the Ginger rhizome into slices. Put into a small pan with one cup of water and bring to a simmer. Cover. Do not bring liquid to a full boil. Let simmer for 10 minutes. Remove Ginger slices. Drink Ginger Tea before each meal and eat the slices. May add lemon and/or honey to taste.

Heartburn

Ginger Tea will also work as a heartburn remedy. Make the tea when experiencing heartburn, then sip slowly.

Migraine

Ginger Tea works to relieve migraine. Make the tea as soon as possible to the onset of the migraine. Sip Ginger Tea slowly.

Colds and Flu

Make Ginger Tea as soon as symptoms occur. Drink Ginger Tea

three times a day for three days.

Menstrual Cramps
Menstrual cramps can be a mild aching to a full-blown debilitating pain. Make Ginger Tea and drink three times a day while cramping.

20

Green Tea

Are you under stress? Have you recently moved, gotten a divorce, suffered the death of a loved one, started back to school, made a job change, or any other major change in your life? If so, you are under stress, even if any of those things were right to do. There are a number of other stresses in life as well, living through a chaotic times, dealing with difficult people, whether co-workers or family. Many things put stress in our lives.

And **stress** can make us sick. So what can we do about it? Drink green tea!

Aside from helping your body deal with stress, Green Tea has been used for:
- Cancer
- Prevent Tooth Decay
- Immune System
- Sunburn
- High Blood Pressure
- Lower Blood Sugar

Cancer
Properties in green tea have been proven to destroy free radicals. It is also full of antioxidants. One in particular, "EGCG," has been

HEALING HERBS FROM YOUR KITCHEN

proven to reduce tumor growth.

Green Tea is a wonderful anti-cancer medication. It can slow, and sometimes even stop, the growth of cancer cells. It has been shown to help defeat lung cancer. Of course that does not mean if you drink Green Tea while you smoke a cigarette you'll be safe. Nothing can cure such stupidity. But Green Tea can be your front line of defense.

Prevent Tooth Decay

Green Tea has antibacterial agents that can keep you healthy. These agents have been known to slow the growth of dental plaque.

Immune System

Because of these agents, drinking green tea stimulates the immune system and fights infection.

Sunburn

Applying it directly to skin after a sunburn can even help rejuvenate skin and promote quicker healing. It will even attack skin cancer cells that may be forming on your skin if you spend a lot of time under the sun.

High Blood Pressure

Green tea is a mild diuretic. As a result it can lower high blood pressure. It helps with high cholesterol too by destroying bad cholesterol and promoting good cholesterol.

I drink green tea every morning with a little lemon. The lemon is good for lowering blood pressure too.

Blood Sugar

Diabetics rejoice. Drinking green tea can lower your blood sugar. Drink 2-3 cups a day for maximum effect.

That is really good news! With so many benefits and only one caution, how can you lose?

One caution: Those with overactive thyroid should be cautious

using green tea.

21

Marjoram

Marjoram is a lightly fragrant herb that, traditionally, is used to season German and Polish dishes. It can be used fresh as a garnish, and added to vegetables. But don't sell Marjoram short. It is also used for sinus conditions and hay fever, indigestion, asthma, colds, coughs, headache, dizziness, and stomach pains.

Marjoram has been used for:

- Microbial Infections (including food poisoning and viruses)
- Indigestion
- Mouthwash and Gargle
- Hay Fever, Sinusitis, Congestion, Asthma, Coughs, Colds
- Digestive Aid
- Antidepressant
- Rheumatism
- Aromatherapy
- Heart Health

Microbial Infections

Marjoram contains antibacterial, antiseptic and antiviral properties. It will address such conditions as food poisoning, and viruses like flu, mumps and measles. It works as a preventative to tetanus. Any time you get a cut, scrape or wound, apply a Mild Marjoram Tea solution to the cut before bandaging.

Marjoram Tea will also work on conditions like malaria (which is a protozoan infection) and typhoid, but the best solution to typhoid is cleanliness. Always boil water 20 minutes before drinking, and keep your environment and your body, especially your hands, clean.

It is also a mild analgesic. So for those who are NSAID sensitive (aspirin-like products, try Marjoram Tea instead.

Mild Marjoram Tea
1 teaspoon dried Marjoram in a cup
Add 1 cup boiling water
Let steep for 10-20 minutes
Can drink 1-4 cups daily
Honey to taste

Indigestion
Make Mild Marjoram Tea. Drink 2 cups over the next two hours slowly.

Mouthwash or Gargle
Make Mild Marjoram Tea, unsweetened, and add a little salt. Cool. Then use as a mouthwash or gargle.

Hay Fever, Sinus Congestion, Asthma, Colds, Coughs
(expectorant)
Drink Mild Marjoram Tea as needed.

Digestive Aid
To increase digestion efficiency, calm the stomach, improve appetite, relieve nausea and excessive gas, address intestinal parasites, relieve diarrhea and intestinal infections, relieve constipation and soothe stomach distress, drink a Mild Marjoram Tea, can drink up to 4 cups daily.

Strong Marjoram Tea, Using Fresh Marjoram
Grind fresh Marjoram into paste.
2-6 teaspoons fresh Marjoram paste
Add 1 cup cold water
Let soak for 24 hours
Strain liquid into cup
Add honey

Antidepressant
Use the strongest recipe (6 teaspoons for each cup of water) as an antidepressant and nervous disorders.

Rheumatism Pain (topical)
Grind fresh Marjoram into a paste
Add hot water and a little oatmeal for consistency
Apply to affected areas

Bath, Aromatherapy, Insomnia
Fresh Marjoram placed in a cheesecloth bag and placed under the tap as you run your bathwater is good for the skin, and helps the body relax.

Heart Health
Marjoram does several things to keep your heart healthy. It prevents the buildup of cholesterol, lowers blood pressure, and aids in improved blood circulation.

How to Grow Marjoram
Although Marjoram is a perennial, it is usually grown as an annual because it does not winter over in cold climates.

Start seeds indoors until all danger of frost is past before transplanting outside.

Make mounds as a border around other plants, and plant the seedlings on top of the mound. As it branches, it will root itself down into the mound, thus creating an attractive border. It also works well in containers, since the stems and leaves drape over the sides of the pot. Marjoram makes a great companion plant to other vegetables, and is a great addition to any garden.

You may dry the leaves in a dark place and store the dried leaves in a dark place to retain flavor.

You may also store Marjoram in vinegar for a refreshing addition to winter greens.

If you are considering growing Marjoram, remember it is cold sensitive. You will need to bring it in inside the winter.

22

Onion

There is a lot of overlap in how herbs work in the body. This is excellent news! It means that when you run out of one herbal family of remedies, you still have access to many others that do the same, or similar, things.

The Onion is no exception. In fact, it contains a host of remedies that heal and prevent illness. Let's look at flavonoids as an example. Onions contain around forty of these health boosters. It used to be, in the nutritional dark ages of the 70s and 80s, flavonoids were considered unnecessary ingredients in a food or herb, especially when the active ingredient was something else. True, flavonoids are not active ingredients. But "active" ingredients need some help in order to work. As it turns out, flavonoids are "activating" ingredients. They facilitate the herb or food to do its work.

One such flavonoid – quercetin – protects the eyes against cataracts, cardiovascular disease, and cancer. As for treating cancer, onion contains twenty-five compounds that inhibit cancerous growths.

The very things that onion is blamed for causing, watery eyes, a burning, runny nose, are also the very things onion can be used to treat. Do you have **sinus congestion**, or a **cold** that is making your eyes water and your throat raw? Breathe in some raw onion fumes.

Onion is also an **antibacterial** and **anti-fungal** agent. This means you can prevent the cold and congestion by regular use of onion, the closer to raw the better.

Onion also helps relieve nausea and other gastrointestinal disorders, including colic in babies. And it strengthens the appetite.

Do you have a problem with high cholesterol? Onion can raise your HDL, or "good" cholesterol up to 30% over time. It also has diuretic properties.

Is the whole neighborhood infected with colds and you haven't caught it yet? Sleep with a cut onion next to your bed at night to prevent viruses.

Other things Onion has been used for:

- Acne
- Earache
- Hemorrhoids
- Coughs and Colds
- Cuts and Wounds

Acne
Squeeze the juice from one onion
Apply with cotton ball to affected area before bed.
In morning, wash face.
Repeat each evening before bed.

Onion Compress, for arthritis and chest congestion
Make an onion compress with cut and boiled onion
Put the boiled onion into a thick cloth and apply to joints for relief.
Or apply to chest to relieve congestion

Earache
Squeeze some onion juice in a bit of cotton ball and put it in the

outside of your ear canal. It literally draws the infection out of your ear. You can even put a drop or two of onion juice inside the ear canal for the same, if not better, effect. This is especially effective for "swimmer's ear," which is a fungal infection.

Hemorrhoids

If no bleeding is present, insert a piece of onion directly into the anus overnight.

If bleeding is present, mix equal parts of onion juice with olive oil and apply to the affected area before bed.

Onion Cough and Cold Medicine Cut

up one onion.
Boil in 1 cup of water for 10 minutes.
Strain through tea strainer or cloth.
Add honey.
Take throughout the day.

Alternative Cough and Cold Medicine

Boil one onion in water with added honey.
Do not strain, but sample throughout the day.

Cuts and Wounds

Apply onion juice mixed with equal parts of olive oil directly to affected area.

Raw Onion

Eat raw onion slice daily:

- ✓ To improve **eyesight**
- ✓ To relieve gas and chronic **stomach distress**
- ✓ To regulate **periods**
- ✓ To relieve **menstrual and uterine pain**

23

Oregano

Oregano has been used in both culinary and as an herbal medicine for thousands of years. The reason is that it's so versatile. In addition to being high in antioxidants, it contains anti-microbial, antiviral, anti-fungal, anti-inflammatory and anti-parasitic properties. In fact, the same amount of antioxidants you'll find in an apple can also be found in a tablespoon of fresh Oregano. Regular use of Oregano inhibits the activities of bacteria and other microorganisms.

Oregano has been used for:
- Acne
- Mouthwash and Gargle
- Sinus Conditions
- Topical Pain Reliever
- Aromatherapy
- Skin Irritations and Dandruff
- Lice
- Asthma
- Earache
- Toothache
- Colds and Flu
- Herpes and Hepatitis

- Yeast Infection
- Food Poisoning and Intestinal Parasites

An herbal tea made with Oregano also helps to address digestive problems, such as flatulence, nausea, headaches, vomiting, diarrhea, urinary problems, lung disorders and jaundice. The tea can also be used as a mouthwash. Oil of Oregano can be used to soothe an infected tooth. Topically, a paste can be made to ease arthritis pain, insect bites, and many skin problems.

Mild Oregano Tea
1 teaspoon dried Oregano
1 cup boiling water
Add water to Oregano leaves, let steep for 10 minutes
Drink Mild Oregano Tea for indigestion, bloating, flatulence, and headaches.

Acne
Before bed, apply Mild Oregano Tea with cotton ball after washing face. In the morning, wash face again, and apply Mild Oregano Tea with cotton ball.

Mouthwash and Gargle
Make Mild Oregano Tea and let cool. Add salt, rinse out mouth or gargle. It also fights plaque and gum disease.

Steam Inhalant, for sinus conditions
Fill pot with water, add a handful of Oregano leaves, and bring to boil.
Place towel over head and breathe in steam.
This helps clear sinuses.

Oregano Paste, for topical pain reliever
Pound Oregano leaves into a paste, with a little tea or water, plus a bit of oatmeal for desired consistency.

Apply topically to swollen joints, such as sprains and rheumatism, swelling, itching, sores and aching muscles. Oregano paste can be used to soothe bee and wasp stings, red ant bites, even venomous spider and snakebites. Oregano is an efficient pain reliever.

Aromatherapy
Oregano can be put into soaps, lotions, oils, steam facials and baths. Oregano Oil can be used for massages.

To make a fragrant bath, put a handful of Oregano leaves into a coffee filter or a mesh bag. Run your bathwater over the bag and allow it to steep with you as you bathe. Don't forget to relax in the warm, fragrant water to soak away sore muscles or the cares of the day.

Skin Irritations and Dandruff
Apply a few drops of Oregano Oil to scalp before bed to defeat dandruff. Shampoo hair in the morning.

Apply Oregano Oil to the skin for irritating conditions such as eczema, and for insect bites.

Lice
Apply Oregano Oil to scalp and let sit for 1/2 hour.
Comb lice out of hair.
Shampoo.
Repeat daily until lice and eggs are all gone.

Asthma
Rub Oregano Oil on chest for healthy vapors whenever needed.

Oregano Oil
Wash fresh Oregano and pat dry. Place on a towel to finish air drying.

Gently pound Oregano sprigs with meat tenderizer on a cutting board to bruise and break plant fibers. Set aside.

Heat 1 cup oil until slightly warm. Pour into clean glass container. Add crushed Oregano.

Cover and put in cool, dark place or refrigerator for 3 days.

Earache
Apply 1-2 drops Oregano Oil to affected ear.

Toothache
With eyedropper, apply a few drops to affected tooth. This will kill the bacteria causing the infection if applied daily.

Colds and Flu
Use 3 drops of Oregano Oil three times a day to ward off colds and flu.

Herpes and Hepatitis
Use Oregano Oil on herpes infections and to help strengthen a body damaged by hepatitis.

Strong Oregano Tea
Wash fresh or dried Oregano leaves, then chop
Put 1 cup chopped Oregano leaves into 4 cups water
Boil for 10-15 minutes
Let steep for 5 minutes
Strain liquid from leaves
Drink 1/2 cup three times a day
Store remainder in glass container for later use.

Drink Strong Oregano Tea for fevers, coughs, urinary infections, bronchial problems, to promote menstruation, diarrhea, vomiting and jaundice.

Yeast Infection
The Strong Oregano Tea Concoction is great to address both vaginal and oral yeast infections. For a vaginal infection, drink the Strong Oregano Tea Concoction three times a day. It's gentler on your body, and gets rid of the infection.

Nursing mothers whose infants have oral yeast infections can both drink the tea and apply some of the tea to their nipples before nursing. Also, use an eye dropper to apply the medicinal tea to the inside of the baby's mouth. It doesn't matter if the infant spits it back out again. The idea is to apply the tea to the affected areas of the infant's mouth.

Toenail Fungus, Fingernail Fungus, Athlete's Foot
Prepare a Strong Oregano Tea Concoction as a soak. Soak for 1/2 hour daily. The concoction can be either warm or cool.

Need Antibiotics?
The latest research is finding that Oregano's antibiotic properties parallel those of streptomycin and penicillin. My grandmother died of pneumonia. An herbal remedy course that included deep breathing an herbal steam plus drinking Strong Oregano Tea Concoction four to six times a day may have saved her life. She was a young woman in her thirties when she died. Best of all, she would not have developed a dependence on Oregano tea the way one does with streptomycin and penicillin.

Food Poisoning, Giardia, Pinworms and other Intestinal Parasites Drink 1/2 cup Strong Oregano Tea Concoction 3 times a day to fight the effects of food poisoning, giardia, pinworms or other intestinal parasites.

24
Parsley

If you grow your own Parsley, you won't fall for poisonous look-alikes, such as fool's parsley, which can be deadly. Parsley piert, another look-alike, is not deadly, and can be used as a healing herb as well.

Parsley has a number of healthful properties, such as an anti-cancer tumor inhibitor, an anti-inflammatory, loaded with anti-oxidants, minerals and vitamins to keep your immune system healthy. It has Vitamin K, which helps build bones and keep them strong. Vitamin K also protects the nerves. It also has properties that help keep your heart healthy.

It has been used for:

- Urinary Tract Infections
- Kidney Stones
- Gastrointestinal Issues
- Headache and Tired Eyes
- Head Lice, Insect Bites, Bee Stings
- High Blood Pressure
- Breath Freshener
- Anti-Cancer Properties

Urinary Tract Infections
Urinary tract infections can be very tenacious and life-threaten-

ing. Your best option is to see your physician. Should a physician not be available then you can try Strong Parsley Tea. Drink one to three cups daily until urine runs clear.

Kidney Stones

Kidney stones can be excruciatingly painful. See your doctor. If one is not available, you may try Strong Parsley Tea. Drink three cups daily until stones pass or symptoms clear.

Strong Parsley Tea, used for kidney stones, bladder infections, and to start **delayed menses**

Wash and dry Parsley root. You may either dry the Parsley root completely and store for later purposes, or use fresh Parsley root.

2 teaspoons of fresh, chopped Parsley root (1 teaspoon dried root)

1 cup boiling water

Pour boiling water over Parsley root.

Let steep 10-20 minutes. Strain into cup.

Sip slowly. Drink 1-3 cups daily.

Note: DO NOT USE IF PREGNANT

Gastrointestinal Issues

Although annoying, gastrointestinal issues are usually not life threatening. A Mild Parsley Tea can be taken. Sip slowly.

 Mild Parsley Tea, used for gastrointestinal disorders, flatulence, indigestion, colic, and as a diuretic

Wash and pat dry Parsley leaves. You may use either fresh or dried Parsley leaves.

2 teaspoons of fresh, chopped Parsley leaves (1 teaspoon dried leaves)

1 cup boiling water

Pour water over Parsley leaves.

Let steep 5-20 minutes. Strain into cup.

Sip slowly for gastrointestinal distress as needed.

Headache and Tired Eyes

Mild Parsley Tea, unsweetened, is an excellent remedy for a headache due to stress. Take a clean rag and dip into a Mild Parsley Tea solution. Wring out excess moisture and apply as a cool dressing for headache and tired eyes.

Lice, Bug Bites, Bee Stings
Dry some Parsley for use during the winter months. Fresh Parsley can be crushed and rubbed directly on a bug bite or bee sting. Otherwise make a Parsley Oil that can be used year around.

Parsley Oil
Wash fresh Parsley (leaves and roots) and pat dry. Place on a towel to finish air drying.

Gently pound Parsley with meat tenderizer on a cutting board to bruise and break plant fibers. Set aside.

Heat 1 cup oil until slightly warm. Pour into clean glass container. Add crushed Parsley.

Cover and put in cool, dark place or refrigerator for 3 days.

Breath Freshener
Chew a few fresh Parsley leaves to freshen breath.

Fresh Parsley
Use fresh Parsley as an addition to cooked vegetables, homemade stews and soups, and scrambled eggs. Although cooking the Parsley won't harm you, you get better nutrition from the raw herb. So add chopped Parsley to everything you cook for added benefit.

High Blood Pressure and Heart Health
Drink 1 cup **Strong Parsley Tea** daily. Also, add fresh Parsley daily to your meals.

Anti-Cancer
This is an excellent herb to use if your body is prone to cancer. Even if it isn't, daily use of Parsley works as a cancer preventative.

Growing Parsley

Parsley is a biennial, meaning it won't produce seeds until the second year. But you can grow it as an annual in cold climates, or grow it inside as a part of your culinary and herbal garden.

Germination is slow, so be patient. To hasten the growth of your Parsley, soak seeds for 24 hours before planting. Water frequently. DO NOT LET THE SEEDS DRY OUT. Parsley requires a lot of sun, so if growing your herb inside, be sure to place under a grow light or in a sunny window.

When growing Parsley outside, remember it makes an attractive companion plant to her herbal garden, as well as a lovely border.

25

Radish

A Healthy Snack

Radishes have an abundance of Vitamin C for their size. They are a healthy low-calorie snack that feeds your body much better than chips which add calories, but steal nutrition. Studies show that a 1/2 cup provides about fourteen percent of your daily need for Vitamin
C.

Do you think that's not enough? Let's take a look at this little package called a radish and compare it to taking a Vitamin C tablet.

The tablet will give you one hundred percent of the daily requirements. Isn't that better that fourteen percent? Not really. If you take a tablet, and your body only needs a portion of the Vitamin C provided, the rest is excreted in your urine. So you've wasted a good portion of the vitamin that your body needs throughout the day. The best way to take Vitamin C, and a number of nutrients as well, is throughout the day.

A radish is a whole package of vitamins, minerals, fiber, and a host of other nutritional aids. So by munching on radishes throughout the day, you feed your body what it needs, throughout the day.

This is the way whole foods work. They aren't refined and isolated, and robbed of what they were designed to do. So eat your radishes, and skip the pills. Vitamin C, a water soluble nutrient, not only is released into the urine if you take more than your body needs, it also needs to be replenished every day. Your body does not store up water soluble nutrients.

A Source of Fiber

Another important part of the humble radish is the amount of fiber it contains. Once again, that half-cup of radishes contains no more than a gram of fiber, not much when you consider your daily dietary needs. But in a fresh salad, you add fiber to a fiber-filled dish, and robust taste besides.

So not only are you feeding your body a whole food, but you're also lowering your risk of diabetes, heart disease, diverticulitis, and cancer. And, speaking of cancer, there are compounds in the radish bulb that can lead to cancer cell death. And since nuclear disasters like that of Fukushima, we need to be aware of what we can do to prevent and kill all the cancer cells possible.

A Note on Healthy Eating

Diet is a four-letter word. A diet implies a temporary solution. That is not what we need. We need to learn how to eat well. The radish is a powerhouse full of nutrition. That same half-cup of radishes only has nine calories. It feeds you, instead of robbing you of nutrition the way chips will do. It's a snack any dieter will appreciate. And it's a food that those who seriously want to learn to eat well can use.

You want foods that feed you, not those that rob your body while it figures out how to digest the stuff you're eating.

Radishes:

- ✓ Work as a detoxifier
- ✓ Keep your liver and stomach in good working order
- ✓ Aid in digestion
- ✓ Cure constipation
- ✓ Work as a diuretic

- ✓ Are low in calories, the perfect snack food
- ✓ Work as a skin soother on insect bites
- ✓ Keep your skin healthy and beautiful
- ✓ Work against jaundice
- ✓ Guard against and treat urinary tract infections
- ✓ Help with weight loss because of high fiber content

CAUTION: Do not eat large quantities of radishes. They can irritate the stomach. They are not good for pregnant women. Radishes are not good for people with gallbladder issues. If you have gall stones, DO NOT EAT RADISHES.

All parts of the Radish are edible, including the leaves. The seeds may be sprouted and then eaten as fresh sprouts on sandwiches and in salads.

Mashed Radish can be used as a facial pack.

Radish Juice is a great facial cleanser and toner.

Growing Radishes

Put them as companion plants between your other vegetables. They protect the rest of your garden from pests.

26

ROSEMARY

Rosemary is an aromatic evergreen that does best in warmer climates. If you plan to grow Rosemary in a cooler climate, make it a part of your indoor herb garden.

As a culinary spice, Rosemary works well in salads, soups, baked vegetable and meat dishes. It also makes a great addition with garlic and sea salt for a sprinkle on eggs, and as an addition to herb breads. Rosemary is a versatile spice.

It has been used for:

- Cancer Prevention
- Anti-Inflammatory and Pain Reliever
- Immune Booster
- Antibacterial
- Digestive Helper
- Diuretic Agent
- Respiration Improver
- Liver Detoxifier
- Aromatherapy
- Hair Growth
- Fresh Breath
- Anti-Aging Skin Health

Cancer Preventative

Research is showing promising results in Rosemary's effects against a number of cancers, including breast cancer, prostate cancer, colon cancer leukemia, and skin cancer.

Anti-Inflammatory and Pain Reliever

Although it isn't the only herb that provides minor pain relief, it is one of them.

Rosemary Tea addresses a number of ailments:

- ✓ Mild pain relief
- ✓ Inflammation
- ✓ Assists immune system
- ✓ Works with digestion
- ✓ Help relieve ulcer pain
- ✓ Respiratory issues, such as coughs and colds, and also works as an expectorant.

Rosemary Tea

1 teaspoon Rosemary
1 cup boiling water
Add water to Rosemary, and let steep 10-20 minutes.
Sip slowly. No more than 1 cup per day. Overuse can irritate the stomach.

CAUTIONS: Pregnant women should not drink Rosemary Tea, since it will cause uterine contractions. And those with high blood pressure should not take Rosemary internally, since it causes a rise in blood pressure.

Topical Uses

Rosemary works both inside and out like an analgesic. For topical relief to swollen joints due to arthritis, strains or sprains, make this Rosemary Lotion:

Rosemary Lotion, also good as an anti-aging cream, as well as for muscle spasms and eczema. Just rub it in. 1 teaspoon Rosemary

ground to a powder 1 cup warm olive oil or grape seed oil.
Mix well.
Apply to sore, aching muscles and joints. Massage in.

Rosemary Liniment, also used for topical pain relief, antibacterial ointment for cuts and abrasions.
1 tablespoon Rosemary, ground to a
powder 1 pint of apple cider vinegar.
Boil gently for about 10 minutes.
Do not strain. Pour liquid into a jar and use as needed.
For external use only.

Aromatherapy

Rosemary has been used for hundreds of years to improve memory. But not only taking Rosemary internally helps. It has also been found that Rosemary in a steam, such as in aromatherapy, can also help. It seems the scent of Rosemary also helps elevate a person's mood at the same time.

For those suffering from migraines:
Boil water in a large pot
Add a small handful of Rosemary
Place a towel over your head, and breathe steam for about 10 minutes.

Hair Growth
1 cup water
1 tablespoon Borax
1 teaspoon Rosemary
Pour mixture over hair after final shampoo rinse

Anti-Dandruff Solution
1 dark bottle (such as an old wine bottle)
2 cups vinegar
Several sprigs of both Mint and Rosemary
Put all ingredients into bottle and cork tightly

Store in dark place for at least a week
Apply a little after every shampoo, and massage into scalp

Mouthwash
2 cups of boiling water
1 tablespoon Rosemary
Let steep for 10 minutes
Strain, cover and store in refrigerator
Rinse mouth daily

27

Sage

Sage is easy to grow, easy to use, and a valuable addition to your medicine chest. Sage has a huge variety of natural properties that include analgesic, antibacterial, anti-cancer, antifungal, antioxidant, astringent, menses starting, nerve calming and system purifying agents.

Although primarily for culinary use, Sage has also been used for:

- Aromatherapy
- Oral Hygiene
- Colds and Sore Throats
- Winter Tonic
- Digestion
- Insect Repellent (including lice)
- Menopause and Extra Heavy Menses
- Memory Enhancer
- Darken Gray Hair

Aromatherapy

Sage is a natural deodorant. You can combine Sage with other herbs for a fragrant bath, or simmer some on your stove to deodorize your home. One way is to make Mild Sage Tea with a little lemon juice. Place in a spritzer bottle to deodorize the home. A Mild Sage without the lemon makes a fragrant body spray, deodorant and after shave.

Mild Sage Tea
1 teaspoon Sage
1 cup boiling water
A little lemon to taste
Pour water over sage, let steep 10-20 minutes, cool.

Oral Hygiene
Sage has both antibacterial and astringent agents.
Male Mild Sage Tea without the lemon. Add a little cider vinegar to make a great mouthwash and gargle.

Colds, Coughs, Sore Throats, Laryngitis, Tonsillitis
Make Mild Sage Tea with the lemon to keep healthy during cold and flu season. If you do get symptoms, gargle at least twice daily until symptoms disappear.

Sage Tea Variation
Add a little lemon, honey, and mint to your Mild Sage Tea recipe. This will make the tea more potent, helping it become a fever reducer as well as an expectorant for coughs. You may also add chamomile to add a calming effect for those who are sick.

Winter Tonic, for bronchial infections and general winter malaise
1/2 teaspoon Sage
1 teaspoon mint
1 teaspoon comfrey
1 teaspoon red clover
2-4 cups boiling water
Honey to taste
Pour boiling water over herbal mix. Let steep 10-20 minutes. Add honey and sip slowly.

Digestion

Drinking Mild Sage Tea daily will help those with chronic digestive complaints.

Insect Repellent, including lice, and fungal infections including ringworm
The following recipe works well on animals too.

Strong Sage Tea, for ringworm and other fungal infections.
1 tablespoon Sage
1 cup boiling water
Pour water over Sage and let steep for 20 minutes or longer.
Strain, soak affected area in solution two times daily. No need to rinse.

Menopause, Hot Flashes, Drying Breast Milk
Sage helps balance estrogen levels in women. As such, it can help with that general feeling of irritability and anxiety some women feel when their estrogen levels are out of balance, such as before or during menses, and during menopause.

PREGNANT WOMEN SHOULD NOT DRINK SAGE TEA, although eating small amounts of sage with a meal will not harm her or the fetus.
Drink Mild Sage Tea, with or without the lemon daily while addressing the issues of menopause, hot flashes, and drying breast milk.

Memory Enhancer
Drink Weak Sage Tea daily to address the issues of Attention Deficit Disorder and cognitive functions.

Darken Gray Hair
Use Strong Sage Tea as a hair rinse. Not only will your hair feel soft and shiny, but it will darken the gray and have it blend in with the rest of the hair better.

If you have naturally very dark hair, you can enhance the darkening effect by boiling black walnut hulls with the Sage and using that water (after straining) as a hair rinse.

If you have naturally light hair, you will not want to use a sage rinse unless you wish to darken your hair.

28

Summer Savory

Summer Savory is an herb that you'll want to grow every year. Find a place with poor soil, the edge of a gravel driveway or a stony slope. Summer Savory does not need to take space in your well-nourished garden.

Use the whole herb, roots, stems and flowers. The most potent parts are the flowering shoots.

Summer Savory has been used for:

- Gastrointestinal Issues
- Diabetic Thirst
- Congestion, Coughs, Sore Throats
- Bug Bites and Bee Stings
- Arthritis
- Antiseptic
- Aromatherapy
- Culinary Herb

Note: Pregnant women should not use Summer Savory

Gastrointestinal Issues

If you have chronic gastrointestinal problems, look at your diet first.

Are you eating too much? Do you have too much sugar in your

diet? Are there certain foods you should be avoiding? As you work through those issues, Mild Summer Savory Tea will help. This tea is also mild enough for infants who suffer from colic.

Mild Summer Savory Tea
1 teaspoon Summer Savory
1 cup boiling water
Pour boiling water over chopped herb. Let steep 5-20 minutes. Sip slowly.

Diabetics
Drink Mild Summer Savory Tea to alleviate excessive thirst.

Congestion, Coughs, Sore Throats
When we get to cold and flu season, we need not be victims of viruses. We have an herbal army ready to fight for us. One such soldier is Sage. You can make Strong Summer Savory Tea for all your cold and flu symptoms, even for diarrhea and as an antiseptic to fight germs lingering around the home.

Strong Summer Savory Tea
1 tablespoon Summer Savory
1 cup boiling water
Honey to taste
Poor boiling water over chopped herb. Let steep 20 minutes. Add honey. Sip slowly

To clean the sick room, add a little vinegar, put in a spray bottle, and use to disinfect all surfaces.

Bug Bites, Bee Stings
Rub fresh Summer Savory on affected area.

Arthritis
Arthritis doesn't affect all people as they age, but those who are affected wish there was something to ease the pain. Summer Savory Ointment works well for arthritic joints. But don't stop

there. It also works on skin irritations.

Summer Savory Ointment

1 cup fresh Summer Savory (or 1/2 cup dried)
2 cups olive oil (or other pure vegetable oil such as safflower oil)
Heat on low heat – DO NOT BOIL – uncovered for 1 hour Cool, strain into bottle with tight cap. Use for irritated skin.

To make a thicker ointment, add 1 to 1/2 ounce beeswax after straining, and heat on same low heat until beeswax melts. Put into jars with tight caps.

Aromatherapy

Place some leaves in a bag to put in your bath for a pleasingly aromatic bath.

Make some Summer Savory steam by boiling leaves in a large pot to scent your home.

Culinary Herb

When making a pot of beans, add some Summer Savory to your pot, or sprinkle some over each serving to reduce flatulence. It also tastes really good!

Add Summer Savory to salads and vegetables too. It blends well with thyme, marjoram and basil. Yumm!

Make an herb vinegar using sprigs of thyme, marjoram, basil and Summer Savory. Save a dark bottle, wash well and dry. Poke the herb sprigs into the bottle. Add cider vinegar, and store in dark place for one month. Then use on salads as part of your salad dressing. Delicious!

How to Grow:

Grow near beans to repel insects. Find your permanent location, and plant, just barely covering the seeds. DO NOT TRANSPLANT. This plant does not like to be disturbed.

In colder climates, cover so that it can winter over. If you are below Zone 5, it may not winter over at all, and you may need to seed it every year as you would an annual.

Its cousin, Winter Savory, may winter over better.

When the plant gets about 6-12 inches tall, and before it flowers, cut the stems, tie into bundles and hang upside down in an open room.
When leaves are dry, remove them, and store them in airtight jars.

Leave some of the plants to flower so that you have a ready supply of Summer Savory for next year. They will probably seed themselves down. Or you can try to harvest the seeds before they fall for your next spring planting.

29

Tarragon

Many herbs, like Tarragon, work to KEEP the body healthy more than they do once the body has become ill. But even so, it's wise to have some Tarragon on hand for when an illness strikes. You are using these herbs regularly for seasoning, right?

Tarragon has been used for:

- Insomnia and Tension
- Headache and Depression
- Toothache
- Digestive Aid
- Hiccups
- Internal Parasites
- Antibacterial
- Heart Health

Insomnia and Tension
For a calming effect before bed, make a Tarragon Tea.

Tarragon Tea
1 Tablespoon fresh Tarragon, or 1 ½ teaspoon dried Tarragon
1 ¾ cup boiling water
Pour water over leaves

Let stand for 40 minutes
Strain into teacup and drink
May drink daily.

Headache and Depression
Handful of dried leaves into 2-3 cups boiling water.
Lean over steam with towel over head and breath in the vapors.

Toothache, adults only
Chew a few leaves and make a paste in mouth.
Hold over infected tooth with tongue for numbing effect.

Digestive Aid
Put a handful of dried leaves in a quart jar.
Add apple cider vinegar.
Let sit for 7 hours.
Take 1 tablespoon before each meal.

Hiccups
Chew a few Tarragon leaves to stop hiccups.

Strong Tarragon Tea for Intestinal Parasites
1/4 cup Tarragon leaves
1 quart boiling water
Pour water over Tarragon leaves.
Let stand for 10 minutes.
Drink 2 cups in morning, and 2 cups in evening until all sign of worms are gone.

Cuts
Crush a few fresh leaves and apply to cut for anti-bacterial effect.
Let sit for 10 minutes,
Then wash and bandage as usual.

Heart Health
Recent studies are showing that Tarragon helps prevent heart attacks and strokes by inhibiting the activating of platelets and the

formation of blood clots in the small blood vessels of the heart and brain.

Cooking with Tarragon

Fresh Tarragon should be washed and patted dry before using. It is added right before serving so that it retains its flavor and nutritional value.

- ✓ Fresh tarragon makes a great addition to a green salad.
- ✓ Both fresh and dried leaves can be added to a marinade to season fish, lamb and poultry.
- ✓ It is a primary ingredient in French béarnaise sauce.
- ✓ It is the seasoning used to make potica, a sweet, nutty rolled Christmas bread.

Growing Tarragon

Tarragon rarely produces fertile seeds. You may propagate Tarragon is by dividing the roots in the early spring. This doesn't always work, so be patient. One way to help your transplants succeed is to grow them under a hand glass until they root down well. This means to save your gallon pickle jars and place them top side down over the newly separated roots. This gives each plant a kind of mini greenhouse so that it can re-establish itself.

You can bring your Tarragon plant inside during the winter if you can guarantee the plant has at least six hours of sun. Tarragon needs a deep pot of at least 12 inches since it has an aggressive root system. If you live in a cold climate, you will need to cover the plants with several inches of mulch to keep the roots from freezing.

When your plants get 6-10 inches tall, you may begin using the leaves. Dried Tarragon should be stored in a dark place, in a tightly sealed container. It keeps for six months.

30
Thyme

When I get a cold, which is rare, it settles in my sinuses and chest. The cold goes away, but the cough remains. One of my problems is that my system produces too much mucous. Perhaps you can identify because you suffer the same complaints when you catch a cold. Thyme also has expectorant properties.

Thyme has been used for:

- Bronchitis and Asthma
- Congestion
- Internal Parasites
- Menstrual Cramps and PMS
- Mouthwash and Tooth Decay Prevention
- Cleaner and Disinfectant
- Wound Disinfectant
- Insect Repellent
- Fungicide

Bronchitis, Asthma Reliever
1 teaspoon thyme, chopped finely
1 teaspoon honey
Mix together and take to soothe the lungs and air passages.
This mixture also works to break a fever, so feel free to use it for someone who is seriously ill.

Relieve Congestion
Put 1 tablespoon of Thyme into a large pot of gently boiling water. Bend over pot with towel draped over head and breathe in steam to help relieve congestion.

Thyme Tea, for internal parasites, menstrual cramps and PMS
1 teaspoon Thyme
1 cup boiling water
Add boiling water to Thyme, set steep for 5-20 minutes
Add a little honey or lemon to taste and sip slowly.
Thyme Tea also helps with digestion by removing excess mucous. Drink Thyme Tea when the day, or the night, has stressed you. It provides a soothing drink after a nightmare, and is safe for children.

Oral Hygiene
Make Thyme tea and let cool. Rinse mouth thoroughly at least once a day.

Household Cleaner and Disinfectant, for house and body Thyme is a natural disinfectant without the harsh chemicals. Thyme has natural anti-microbial properties.

Thyme Cleaner, also good for a sick-room spray
2 cups boiling water
1 tablespoon Thyme
Pour water over Thyme, let cool completely.
Add 1 teaspoon dishsoap and strain into clean spray bottle.
Spray onto all hard surfaces and wipe clean with damp cloth that has no added soap.

A Note on Soap:
You won't need more than a teaspoon of liquid soap for this cleaner. Dish soap works well, but it is also loaded with harsh chemicals. If you are sensitive to these chemicals, don't add the soap at all. Soap works because it makes water wetter. It cuts oils

and makes them easier to wipe up. The Thyme Cleaner and Disinfectant works with or without soap.

If you must use a powdered soap or a grated bar soap, dissolve it in the hot mixture before straining it into a spray bottle.

Wound Disinfectant, to prevent infection to wounds, scrapes and cuts
Make Thyme Cleaner and Disinfectant.
Pour 1/2 cup into small bowl.
Add 1 teaspoon honey, and mix well.
Clean wound with solution and clean cloth.

Food Preservative
Sprinkle crushed Thyme over leftovers to make them last longer, and it adds great flavor besides.

Potpourri, Insect Repellent
Add Thyme to your favorite mixture of scented ingredients, such as rose petals, lavender, rosemary, and so on. Put into sachet bags, and store in your undergarments to make them always smell fresh, and in with your blankets and stored clothing to keep insects out.

Also, if you plant Thyme in with your other herbs and vegetables, you naturally repel garden insects, while attracting bees.

Insect Repellent Rub
1 cup boiling water
1 tablespoon Thyme
Add boiling water to Thyme
Let stand until cool.
Strain.
Use equal parts of Thyme mixture with olive oil or other pure vegetable oil (castor oil works for this) Whisk together until creamy.
Place in a jar and store in dark place.

Apply to skin to repel insects.

Fungicide
1/2 cup fresh Thyme
1 cup vinegar (or vodka)
Combine, and let sit for at least 12 hours.
Apply to affected area.

Thyme Poultice, for sore muscles and muscle spasms
Mash fresh Thyme leaves into a paste, or use dried Thyme with a little water or olive oil to make a paste. Apply to affected area and let sit for half an hour, or longer as needed.

Growing Thyme
Thyme is one of the best things you can do for your garden. It is a perennial that has a bush and a creeping variety. It thrives in warm, sunny parts of the garden. It can be grown from seed, or by cuttings, but it does not do well in temperatures that drop below 10 degrees in the winter. If this is your area, you'll want to bring a few plants inside to winter over.

Trim your Thyme back after it flowers to prevent it from becoming woody. You may either dry or freeze your clippings to use later in the year.

31

Tomato

Those of you who garden already know the value of having several tomato plants in your garden. One year, since our backyard was all concrete, we made a huge four foot by four-foot garden box made with 2 x 12 boards. We planted one tomato plant in the center, and various vegetables all around it. I made the dirt by using 1part Perlite, 1part compost, and 1part peat moss.

That tomato plant literally took over the garden. It was five feet high and six feet in diameter. We harvested over a bushel of tomatoes off that one plant.

That was the year we ate all the tomatoes we wanted, and dried the rest. I still made fried green tomatoes besides. We dried enough tomatoes to last us the next two years.

THAT'S the kind of plant to have! And I didn't even have a back yard that I could dig in, just a concrete patio!

Tomatoes have been used for:
- Weight Control
- Overall Immunity
- Heart Disease

- Osteoporosis
- Reduce High Blood Pressure
- Prevent Cancer
- Prevent Diarrhea
- Liver Health
- Skin Cleanser and Revitalizer
- Heal Sunburn

Weight Control

What are the things that people consume to keep their weight under control? Low calorie foods, foods rich in fiber, vitamins and minerals, foods that suppress appetites are what most of us consider. Tomatoes have all of that, and more. The "more"? Tomatoes feed your body while so many "health" foods do not. Tomatoes are a whole food, meaning they contain a whole package of nutrition, not just one or two "diet" advantages.

Overall Immunity

Tomatoes are rich in many nutrients, especially Vitamin C, which is necessary for cell health. Why take a vitamin tablet, when your body needs the whole food? So eat a Tomato a day, and add chopped or sliced Tomatoes to other meals as well. Have you ever had Tomato slices for breakfast, or chopped Tomatoes over eggs in the morning? Delicious!

Heart Disease

Tomatoes are one food that contains more antioxidants after cooking than before. This is good news for those who like spaghetti sauce, chili, lasagna, and other rich tomato dishes. Tomatoes also reduce high cholesterol and keep blood sugars level. So, antioxidants and lower cholesterol, what heart wouldn't fall in love with this terrific food?

Osteoporosis

Part of the cause of osteoporosis is that as a person gets older, the body no longer absorbs nutrients the way it used to. So if you're over fifty, you need extra nutrition to keep your body healthy. Along with a diet high in calcium and Vitamin D, the antioxidants in Tomatoes help shield your bones from damage. Keep those bones healthy! Eat Tomatoes!

High Blood Pressure

The way tomatoes work is that they are able to dissolve animal fat that can clog up artery walls. They are also high in potassium. It's not salt that's the problem with high blood pressure. It's the fact that the salt causes problems when there isn't enough potassium in the diet. So if you increase your potassium, you can still enjoy small amounts of salt.

Maybe it's a good idea to keep a tomato plant inside all year. They grow in greenhouses. Why not inside a home?

Low Blood Pressure Tomato Salad

2 ripe tomatoes, chopped Sprinkle with:
1 teaspoon ground tarragon
1 teaspoon paprika
1 teaspoon ground turmeric
1 teaspoon basil
Dressing: 1 tablespoon lemon juice
Yumm!

Prevent Cancer

Studies are showing that those who eat lots of tomatoes tend to have a lower risk of cancer. This is due to be something called lycopenes. Lycopenes are bioflavonoids related to beta carotene. But is the act of cooking the tomatoes that releases the fat-soluble nutrient.

A fat-soluble nutrient is one that dissolves in fat, which means it can be stored in fatty cells in the body. But you will need a small amount of added oil to release these bioflavonoids. That bit of olive oil that you add to Italian dishes will do the trick.

Stop Diarrhea Tomato Tea
Grind dried Tomato slices (about 12 slices) into powder.
Add 2/3 cup of warm water to dried Tomato powder.
Drink as needed.
OR:
Add dried Tomato powder to warm apple juice, if preferred.
OR:
Add 1 tablespoon dried Tomato powder to small (4 oz.) glass of milk. Drink every 2 hours, as needed.

Liver Health
If you have been diagnosed with liver damage, drinking Tomato juice daily can help restore the liver. Or eat a Tomato a day, if you prefer.

Skin Cleanser and Revitalizer
Ever heard of a Tomato Mask? Well, this is a first for me too.

Tomato Mask
Cut VERY thin slices of Tomato.
Place the slices all over your face and lie down for 10-20 minutes.
Rub some of the Tomato into your skin, then remove all residue, but do not rinse your face.

This works as an exfoliate and skin conditioner, and the acid in the Tomato will restore your PH balance.

Tomato Scrub, for acne skin
Rub slices of Tomato directly into the skin, concentrating on blemished areas. Wipe off, but no need to rinse.

Caution: Tomato can become an irritant if used too frequently. Use both the Tomato Mask and the Tomato Scrub no more than twice a week.

Sunburn
Soak Tomato slices in buttermilk. Apply to sunburned areas. Let

sit from 10-20 minutes. Remove and rinse.

32

Turmeric

Turmeric is not only used as a culinary spice, it has also been used as a dye in India for over 2500 years. It is also used as a natural antiseptic and antibacterial agent for cuts and burns. It may also work for other skin conditions such as psoriasis.

Turmeric has been used for:

- Cancer
- Memory Enhancer
- Anti-Inflammatory
- Hearth Health
- Blood Sugar
- Toothpaste
- Tinted Moisturizer
- Soap
- Dandruff
- Fabric Dye

Cancer

Cauliflower seasoned with Turmeric prevents prostate cancer, and can even stop the growth of prostate cancer that already exists. As a cancer fighter, it slows the growth of breast cancer, reduces the risk of Leukemia, and prevents skin cancer.

Memory Enhancer

It is also believed to enhance memory and treat Alzheimer's, and to alleviate the symptoms of Parkinson's disease. Those who have been on simvastatin for a long time run the risk of developing Parkinson'slike symptoms once they stop taking simvastatin. With Turmeric capsules, you can solve the problem of high cholesterol as well as address this unwarranted side-effect.

Anti-Inflammatory

It has anti-inflammatory properties, but is also a NSAID. People sensitive to NSAIDs, such as aspirin, Aleve, ibuprofen, and the rest, need to understand that while using Turmeric as a pain killer may help with no side-effects, you may be sensitive to Turmeric as well. That said, because it also has the added ability to detoxify the liver, it may be safe to use even for those sensitive to NSAIDS. The reason is one of the side effects of prescription and over the counter NSAIDS is its damage to the liver. And in that respect, Tylenol is no better.

Because it has a strong, and to some, and unpalatable flavor, those who choose to use Turmeric as a medicine can purchase clear capsules and fill them with Turmeric powder.

CAUTION: DO NOT USE TURMERIC IF YOU HAVE GALLSTONES OR BILE OBSTRUCTION ISSUES.

Turmeric increases the production of bile, so it is good for the digestion in most people. But if you have an ulcer or a sensitive stomach, you will want to avoid Turmeric.

Heart Health

Turmeric is good for your heart. It reduces "bad" cholesterol (HDL levels) and increases "good" cholesterol (LDL levels) in the blood.

If you take Turmeric in capsule form, although studies are not complete, no negative side effects have been noted, and even taking as much as 12 grams per day have not shown adverse effects.

Blood Sugar

Turmeric lowers blood sugar. This is good news for diabetics who are looking for natural ways to control their blood sugar levels.

Other Uses for Turmeric:

Toothpaste

Add a little to your toothpaste as a whitening agent. Although Turmeric stains everything yellow, the short amount of time it will be on your teeth actually whitens them.

Tinted Moisturizer

Do you use tinted moisturizer instead of foundation? If your skin is more golden than pink, try a little Turmeric in your moisturizer to brighten your skin.

Soap

If you make your own soap, you may want to add some Turmeric for its lovely yellow color as well as how it makes your skin feel.

Dandruff

Apply a mixture of Turmeric and your favorite oil, such as olive or coconut oil, and apply to your scalp. Massage it in. Let sit for 15 minutes longer, then shampoo as usual. It gets rid of dandruff!

Turmeric Tea, for a long, healthy
life Boil water in a quart pan.
Add 1 teaspoon Turmeric powder.
Let simmer for 10 minutes, then strain.
Add ginger and/or honey to taste.
Drink daily.

Fabric Dye

Bring a pot of water to a boil.
Add 3 tablespoons of Turmeric.
Let simmer for at least 10 minutes.

Add fabric, such as white tee-shirts you want tie-dyed.
Add Turmeric to Your Play Dough Recipe

And Lastly...Color Easter Eggs Bright Yellow
Add Turmeric to your homemade play dough for a bright yellow dough.

Naturally color Easter eggs with Turmeric for a lovely yellow color.

Books by Mama Prepper

39 Healthy Teas You Can Make at Home
Your Herbal Garden
Healthy Herbs from Your Kitchen
Mama's Medicines – Growing Your Backyard Apothecary

DEDICATION

This book is dedicated to all those who want to do more for their bodies and their health.

ACKNOWLEDGMENTS

My husband provided me the time and space to turn this work into a reality. My children have always been my fans. Lisa is an inspiration as well as a great beta reader. Patsy is a terrific proof reader, and
And a big thanks to all my friends who cheer me on.

DISCLAIMER

The herbal articles are for entertainment and educational purposes only. The author is not a physician, and the contents of these articles should not be viewed or taken as medical advice. The views expressed are the opinion of the author and should not be taken as an endorsement of any product or practice. Herbs can and do interact with pharmaceuticals. No herb or herbal product should be taken without consulting a qualified physician. The author disclaims any liability arising directly or indirectly from the use of the information of any product, plant or practice mentioned herein.

ABOUT THE AUTHOR

An unfortunate series of financial setbacks left her nearly destitute. She couldn't even afford the gas to go into town to see her doctor. She was no longer young. How was she to stay healthy if she couldn't order her meds? She began to do research on alternative medicine.

What she found totally amazed her. She discovered a whole world of herbal medicine that completely changed her life. As she learned to make her own meds, she began to realize how the pharmaceutical industry had been keeping her sick.

Now she shares her knowledge with others, providing the opportunity for each one of us to be healthier than Big Pharma intended.

ISBN-10: 1495909409
ISBN-13: 978-1495909405